Veterinary Healthcare Services | *Options in Delivery*

Veterinary Healthcare Services

Options in Delivery

Thomas E. Catanzaro, DVM, MHA, FACHE

Thom Haig, DVM

Peter Weinstein, DVM, MBA

Judi Leake, DVM

Heather Howell, RVT, MBA

Iowa State University Press / Ames

Thomas E. Catanzaro, DVM, MHA, FACHE, Diplomate, American College of Healthcare Executives, is the first veterinarian to receive board certification with the American College of Healthcare Executives. He has spent the last decade building the largest veterinary-exclusive, diplomate-led veterinary consulting team in the United States. His full-time consultation and seminar schedule has given him knowledge and appreciation for the multitude of practice options.

Thom Haig, DVM, is a partner in a multispecies veterinary hospital in Nevada. He has been a lead consultant for Catanzaro & Associates for the last seven years. He is also co-editor of the VIN practice management board. His past experience with the Nevada State Board brings a unique perspective to the value of medical records.

Peter Weinstein, DVM, MBA, is a veterinarian and hospital administrator at an animal hospital in a suburban setting in southern California. His practice management consultation with Catanzaro & Associates and his experience with state and local veterinary medical associations have provided tremendous exposure to a variety of practice styles.

Judi Leake, DVM, used the lessons from practice management principles of Dr. Catanzaro to allow her to begin an early retirement. Retirement was short-lived, and she is currently building a state-of-the-art hospital and pet resort near Aspen, Colorado.

Heather Howell, RVT, MBA, is a hospital administrator in a seven-doctor, mixed animal practice in Nevada. Her interests in human resources and personnel management contribute to the team-building emphasis of this book.

Iowa State University Press
2121 South State Avenue, Ames, Iowa 50014

Orders: 1-800-862-6657
Office: 1-515-292-0140
Fax: 1-515-292-3348
Web site: www.isupress.edu

First edition, 2000

Library of Congress Cataloging-in-Publication Data

Veterinary healthcare services: options in delivery/Thomas E. Catanzaro ... [et al.].
    p. cm.
  ISBN 0-8138-0929-0
  1. Veterinary medicine—Practice. I. Catanzaro, Thomas E.
  SF756.4.V44 1999
  636.089′068—dc21   99-059177

The last digit is the print number: 9 8 7 6 5 4 3 2 1

Contents

Foreword

When I wrote the three volumes of *Building the Successful Veterinary Practice: Leadership Tools* (Volume 1), *Programs & Procedures* (Volume 2), and *Innovation & Creativity* (Volume 3), I integrated team building and leadership into each text. It is my sincere belief that veterinary healthcare teams, not individual providers or astute practice managers, are the keys to success in the new millennium. Therefore, a nuts-and-bolts text was required to provide additional options to the ones provided in the first series of texts.

If I was to "walk the talk," I had to expand the perspective of the approach. How better to do that than to involve active clinicians who are using many of the basic principles of the first series and to have them be the principal authors. The preface that they offer is their idea of the task ahead. As you may note, they are "real" and "honest" clinicians, and I trust them with my reputation, with the clients of our consulting practice and, more importantly, with presenting the changes needed in the veterinary profession.

Thomas E. Catanzaro, DVM, MHA, FACHE
Diplomate, American College of Healthcare Executives

Preface

All of the authors struggled over the title name, searching for something that would seem meaningful to the potential purchaser. The way we came up with this title demonstrates the variety of our team and the irreverence that Tom Cat tolerates in developing such a team. We wanted *Practice Management for the Practicing Veterinarian* and other equally nebulous names. Tom Cat made no suggestions, but he did veto the earlier titles as too general. We credit Peter with starting the process that came to our working title, *Plain English Translations of the Works of Tom Cat*. Those of you who have followed Tom Cat's writings in texts or periodicals instantly know what we mean; he is the most plagiarized author in our profession today. Tom is light years ahead of the traditional "management gimmick" veterinary consulting services and has dedicated himself, his consulting firm, and us to raising the bar and taking the high road of quality healthcare delivery by skilled and trusted healthcare teams. Heck, he is even training veterinary editors that "healthcare" is one word when used as an adjective! At seminars and on the phone, Thom Haig prides himself in speaking three languages—English, German, and Catanzaro.

We pride ourselves in our ability to translate the integrated theory and principles that Tom Cat offers into workable practice solutions and tailoring those solutions to specific practices and their unique needs. As his most faithful translators, the co-authors want to dedicate this book with the utmost irreverence to Dr. Tom Cat. The final title is an extension of our ShirtSleeves Seminars series. In that series Thom and Peter provide the participants with options of different applications of Tom Cat's theories. Thom, Heather, Peter, and Judi all practice in dramatically different environments. They all interpret Tom Cat's theories in their own way. The purpose of this text is to show you the many different ways that these theories can be successfully applied.

Thom Haig, DVM
Peter Weinstein, DVM, MBA
Judi Leake, DVM
Heather Howell, RVT, MBA

List of Abbreviations

ACL—Anterior cruciate ligament
ACT—Activated clotting time
AIDA—Attention, interest, desire, action
a.k.a.—Also known as

b.i.d.—Twice a day

CBC—Complete blood count
CCU—Critical care unit
CD—Compact disc
CE—Continuing education
CHF—Congestive heart failure
CT—Computerized tomography
CTD—Circling the drain
CWT—Per hundred weight

DT—Dental technician
DTM—Dermatophyte Test Media

ECG—Electrocardiogram
EKG—Electrocardiogram
ER—Emergency room

FeLV—Feline leukemia virus
FES—Functional electrical stimulation
FHO—Femoral head ostectomy

HIW—How it works

ICU—Intensive care unit
IOP—Intraocular pressure

IRS—Internal Revenue Service
ISUP—Iowa State University Press
IT—Intake technician
IVM—Ivermectin

J.D.I.—Just do it!

KCS—Keratitis sicca

MRI—Magnetic resonance imaging
MPL—Medial luxating patella
MSDS—Material safety data sheets

NOAH—AVMA's Internet network

OFA—Orthopedic Foundation for
    Animals
OHE—Spay (ovariohysterectomy)
OPN—Outpatient nurse
O.R.—Operating room
OSHA—Occupational Safety and Health
    Administration

PCV—Packed cell volume
PE—Physical Exam
PRN—As needed
QBC—type of automated estimated CBC
    (IDAXX)
q.i.d.—Four times daily

RC—Recovered client

RP—Recovered pet
Rx—Prescription

SA—Surgery assistant
s.i.d.—Once daily
ST—Surgery technician
STT—Schirmer Tear Test
Sx—Surgery

TA—Treatment assistant
TGH—To go home
t.i.d.—Three times a day
TKO—To keep open

TPO—Triple pelvic osteotomy
TPR—Temperature, pulse, and
    respiration

UA—Urinalysis
U/A—Urinalysis
USDA—U.S. Department of Agriculture

V.A.L.—Brand name of Ft. Dodge
    Vitamin Syrup
VIN—Veterinary Information Network
VIP—Very important pet

Veterinary Healthcare Services | *Options in Delivery*

The Era of Revenue Generation— The Front Door Must Swing

1

The secret to an effective veterinary practice does not lie in "one best way." This statement will likely upset the management junkies of the veterinary profession, but will come as, "Yes, so what is your point?" to the majority of veterinary hospital directors. In *Building the Successful Veterinary Practice*, the recent three-volume reference set published by Iowa State University Press, the foundation was laid for the veterinary healthcare delivery approach needed to prosper in the new millennium. The consistent elements in every practice are:

- Consistent Mission Focus
- Inviolate Core Values
- Training to Trust
- Clear Outcome Expectations
- Effective Use of Veterinary Extenders

So in this how-to primer, we will assume that you believe in developing a team approach to the delivery of quality veterinary healthcare services. We will assume that you believe a veterinary practice only sells peace of mind, and clients are allowed to buy from two "yes options" for the quality care needed by the patient. We will assume that you realize a doctor clipping a leg, doing a t.i.d., or even doing 70 percent of the recalls is a doctor wanting to earn about $10 per hour; these are veterinary extender duties! And lastly, we will assume that you understand and embrace the 14 leadership skills of Volume 1 (*Leadership Tools*), the outpatient/inpatient nurse technician of Volume 2 (*Programs & Procedures*), and the learning organization offered in Volume 3 (*Innovation & Creativity*).

We will frequently refer to forms presented in these three volumes, especially Volume 2. Although examples will be provided in this text, the full form or program will not be reproduced. From here forward Vol. 2 will be the only reference to these materials. As a how-to text for the practitioner, there will not be references to other current literature, nor would they be appropriate. This book is intended as a hands-on primer for application of the cutting edge principles presented in the first series.

With all these assumptions, what is left? The answer is options! Alternatives to what you have always done! New looks at old habits (e.g., redesign the paradigm)! Or as our clients (we call them *consulting partners*) often say, "More fun!" Yes, it is possible to put fun back into your practice ... we do it every day!

So in this text, you will not get the "why" that was integrated into the *Building the Successful Veterinary Practice* series; that is where the foundation was laid. We want to provide *options, alternatives,* and, more importantly, *barrier busting ideas*—examples and concepts that will assist the average practice, the growing practice, and the already prospering practice.

Measuring Success by Average Client Transaction (ACT) Rates

There are many current journals and many practice consultants who measure success in practices by quoting the current Average Client Transaction, or the practice gross. We are one of the few professions or small businesses who operate with only income as a measure. Most everyone else in the world understands that net income, not gross, is a key measure of success. This means you must know the expense, or at least know income as an operational ratio. We discussed the diagnostic ratio for doctors and the Travel/Circle Sheet 3 R's (recall—recheck—remind) for next visit planning in Vol. 2, so now appears to be the time to discuss the ACT.

Here is the real question:

In 1997, the ACT was $74. There was a 7 percent medical inflation rate between 1997 and 1998. In 1998, the ACT was $74. Which was a better year for practice income? Please, 1997 or 1998? Choose!

The rest of the story is simply a measure of client visits. In 1997, when the average client transaction was $74, there was one visit per client per year, but in 1998, when the ACT was still $74, there were three visits per year per client! Now which was a better year? Change your mind? Trick question? Okay, try this one:

In 1997, with three visits per client per year, the ACT was $74. There was a 7 percent medical inflation rate between 1997 and 1998. In 1998, when the ACT was still $74, there were still three visits per year per client. Which was a better year for practice income? Please, 1997 or 1998? Choose!

The rest of the story is simply a description of the operational philosophy. In 1997, there were 1.2 doctor hours and 0.9 staff hours spent per client visit, but in 1998, when the ACT was still $74, there were 0.3 doctor hours and 0.5 staff hours per client visit! Now which was a better year? Change your mind? Trick question?

No. These are not trick questions. You saw immediately that the gross dollars of the ACT had very little bearing on the success assessment for these practice situations. If you saw the real answers that fast here, why have you continued to pursue the ACT on a daily basis? It is return visits and higher density scheduling that will make the veterinary practice of the future successful. That is the success question you must resolve now.

Everyone agrees the needs within veterinary practices have changed over the last few decades. No longer can you just hang out a shingle and guarantee success. No longer are there dozens of people lined up outside your door willing to wait for you. We must now extend our beliefs from the *practice* of veterinary medicine to the *business* of veterinary medicine.

As you think about your business you can blame countless challenges outside your door. However, to blame is to abdicate accountability for solutions, and you frequently miss the solutions that can be found within your four walls. The answer to not enough transactions and not enough net can be found by a smarter approach to your current most valuable asset—your client base. This approach includes medical record audits (see Volume 3); better use of your medical record system; and offering programs, protocols, and bundles of services to your pet-owning population.

What Are Programs, Protocols, and Bundles?

Programs are all-inclusive approaches to a single aspect of veterinary medical care. Programs include the marketing of, for example, a dental care program. Programs include the protocols to be followed medically, the tracking and measuring of the results, and the training of the paraprofessionals to implement the program (see Figure 1.1).

Do you see how this program can be used? It is the basis for staff education on the expectations of the practice. This program will establish in both the staff's and client's minds the wellness items for a puppy that are deemed necessary by this practice. The program sheet may be used as a referral sheet for the receptionist, laminated and placed in the exam room for the outpatient nurse (OPN) and doctor, or placed on letterhead to become a client handout.

Here is an example of a program work sheet for a puppy:

Program for: PUPPY

ITEM	REG. CHG	VISIT 1 6-8 weeks	VISIT 2 9-12 weeks	VISIT 3 13-15 weeks	VISIT 4 6-18 weeks
PE/Consult		•		•	
DHPPC		•	•	•	•
Bordetella		•			
Lyme				•	•
Rabies					•
Fecal		•			•
Deworm		•	•	•	•
Rx Sentinel		•			
Weight		•	•	•	•
Behavioral Consult		•			•
Set up Neuter					•
DISCOUNT					
FREE GOODS					
COST TO CLIENT					

FIGURE 1.1

See Appendix 1 for more program work sheets and some examples.

Protocols are outlined lists of medical procedures to be followed when addressing specific sets of clinical signs, confirmed diagnoses, or surgical procedures. The protocol may include everything from radiographs and catheters to lab work and injections. It may be organized for use as an estimate, a treatment list for a staff member, or an education tool for a client. It should include information about what to do at home and any follow-up care needed. Here is an example of a protocol for a minor abscess:

Abscess—minor
  ✓ Office call (veterinary visit, consultation)
  ✓ Isoflurane (first 20 minutes)
  ✓ Drain tube(s)
  ✓ Amoxicillin 15 ml liquid
  ✓ Chlorhexi-Derm flush 4 oz.
  ✓ Amoxi—inject
  ✓ ECG monitoring
  ✓ Standard O.R. setup
  ✓ Preanesthetic screen
  ✓ Minor SURGICAL PACK
  ✓ Induce anesthesia
  ✓ Hospitalization

See Appendix 2 for an extensive list of protocols to stimulate discussion in your practice.

Bundles are computer-generated groupings of those procedures performed for specific conditions. A bundle is linked together so that with a minimal number of keystrokes it can be used to generate an estimate or even an invoice. You can see how the above protocol can easily be stored in your computer to become an estimate as a bundle. It should include links for follow-up care, and the fees should be adjusted as individual line items are adjusted on the fee schedule.

Besides the use of Appendixes 1 and 2 to generate discussion, how do you form the protocols to generate the programs that make the bundles in your computer? One simple method is to print two copies of every recurring medical case for the next several months. Make copies, distribute to the doctors and staff, and discuss one or two at each doctor and staff meeting. Is this the level of medicine we want? Do you treat your pyometras this way? Which of the 3 R's do we need to follow up this type of case? After the master program is in place, continue to add new cases as they occur. In no time at all you'll exceed

Appendix 2, and it will be your hospital's program, not ours. Finally, every new associate should be presented with a copy of your protocols to review *and* comment. They will bring new ideas to your practice and raise the level of care. Possibly most important, by accepting their contributions, you make the programs theirs, too!

The 3 R's—Rechecks, Recalls, Reminders

Our existing client base is our most valuable asset because it is just that, existing! It should be our goal to retain these clients as long as they have pets and are alive or living in the neighborhood. The competition is fierce for the pet owners who don't have a regular veterinarian. So, why not take advantage of what you already have and work aggressively to maintain, nurture, coddle, educate, schmooze, etc. your clients. When selling a practice, the value is very much determined by the quality of your clientele in both goodwill and blue-sky measurements. So, what can you do to nurture these clients and encourage their visits? Communicate, communicate, and communicate!

Every time that the phone rings or the door swings you have a client contact. Each client contact must generate some form of follow-up communication.

Phone Calls

A phone call is a call to action and request for help, whether it's to make an appointment or inquire about a hospitalized animal. A phone call should lead to:

- ✓ booking an appointment,
- ✓ answering a question and sending a brochure or other follow-up information about the practice,
- ✓ offering information about the costs for a particular service and explaining the details of that procedure before offering the price,
- ✓ directing a call to an appropriate staff member to answer a medically oriented question, or
- ✓ creating a computer-generated reminder about the need for a service, product, or future appointment.

Through the years, most veterinarians have developed advanced degrees in expense control. Ask any practitioner what percentage of gross is spent on advertising or maintenance and most can tell you within percentage points. On the other hand, ask most practitioners what percentage of their gross revenues came from in-house diagnostic testing, and you would get a blank stare.

For years when the phone stopped ringing and the door stopped swinging, the pennies got pinched so tight that they screamed. So we added overpriced software and computers to create reminders and help us keep track of our daily receipts. Some developed ways to make their colleagues look bad so that they could look good and with that hopefully steal away their competitor's clients. When none of that worked, we discounted. We prostituted ourselves. We sold out. Now, as we wallow in a world of low-cost vaccination and spay-neuter clinics, we wonder, what went wrong?

Finally, we spent hours at CE meetings with other veterinarians comparing ACT as if the higher the ACT the more successful the practitioner. Wrong!

We have reached the new millennium and it is time for a new philosophical approach. Our goal is to win over clients, nurture them, educate them, and encourage them to invite others to join the family as happy members of our practice. Our goal is to encourage clients to keep coming back as frequently as possible to utilize our services. I would prefer four visits at $50 per visit to one at $150. The goal is client retention. Once you have a client bonded to your practice, they are married to you for as long as you continue to care!

So, what's the trick to increased visits? The 3 R's.

Recall—Recheck—Remind

Every client entering and exiting your practice requires one of the above after their visit to ensure their next visit. Many are simple recalls about the progress of the pet. Others are more elaborate combinations of computer-generated reminders and phone calls or letters. Whatever the case, no one leaves the practice until they are assigned one or more of the 3 R's for computer and staff follow-up.

Office Visit

Let's use an example of a typical office visit consultation to show how to use the computer and the paraprofessional staff that we have to enhance our contacts with a client.

Scenario

Mrs. Gerber and Baby are in for their annual visit with Dr. Haig. Baby needs her annual booster vaccinations, flea control products, and heartworm test, and she has an ear infection.

Upon completion of the office visit/consultation, one or more of the three forms of communication must be generated.

Recheck

If the medical condition of the animal has yet to be cured or the problem remains unsolved, a follow-up visit should be scheduled. A client is not licensed to make the assessment that the dog's ear infection is cleared up. Although most clients feel that they have medical degrees, it is our responsibility to monitor the well-being of the pet until the problem is solved or all the needs fulfilled.

Rechecks should be scheduled prior to departure of the pet and client. Dr. Haig has marked "Recheck 10d" on the travel sheet. This stimulates the following from the receptionist:

> "Mrs. Gerber, Dr. Haig would like to recheck Baby's ears in 10 days. That is the 27th. How is 10:00 a.m. or would 3:00 p.m. be better?" Recommend that Mrs. Gerber book the appointment even if she doesn't know her schedule and then offer, "I will call you later today or tomorrow to confirm that the date and time are OK." Give a refrigerator card with the date and time. "I'll speak to you later Mrs. Gerber and we look forward to ensuring that Baby's ear infection is all better."

Recall, a.k.a. Callbacks

Mrs. Gerber has left. Baby went home with ear medications. Baby has a follow-up appointment scheduled for the 27th. Her fecal and heartworm test results were not finished at the time of their departure. Here is where the recall comes in.

Later that day, Vickie, Dr. Haig's technician, calls Mrs. Gerber, "Congratulations, Baby has passed both her fecal test and heartworm test with flying colors. Remember it is important to stay on that preventative year-round in this area. We will recheck these tests again next year."

What else can be done to impress the socks off Mrs. Gerber? Well, Dr. Haig marked "Recall—3d" on the travel sheet. How about calling her back to find out how Baby's ears are doing after a few days on the medication? How about asking if Mrs. Gerber has any questions or if she is having any difficulty in medicating Baby? Don't forget the re-

·ceptionist promised to call in a day or two to ensure the recheck appointment was convenient. How about calling her 24–48 hours before her recheck appointment to remind her of the appointment? All of these add value to the services you provide. By utilizing the systems in your computer to automatically remind staff and doctors, these important added values are not dropped through the cracks.

Who, What, When, Where, How

Recalls are one of the biggest practice builders ever created. Everyone not doing them either says that they take too long or they are hard to get started. Train the staff to a level of competency and trust, then J.D.I. (Just do it!!!) You'll be amazed by the results. At least weekly, a client says, "My own doctor never called me. Can I come to see you, too?" This is something you should just do. There is no expense involved. You already have the personnel paid to be there. There are times during the day they are looking for things to do. Here is one thing they can do that will be returned to you in tremendously increased perceived value.

Here's the routine:

Either the doctor marks the time on the travel sheet or there is already a computer linkage to a specific time frame for a callback to be made. Each morning, without fail, the receptionist prints out a recall list for that day by name of technician, doctor, or receptionist to make the appropriate type of recall. It can also be at lunch or at the end of the day for the following day. It makes no difference when, as long as it's done daily and someone or some job position is specifically accountable for the task.

Who should make these calls, when should they be made, the scripts used to make them, and the tracking of the calls needs to be decided in advance. Although Vol. 2 offered some scripts, here are some more ideas:

The exam room technician should follow up with any clients for which they did the check-in and/or release. This includes any simple lab work results (e.g., heartworm test, fecal, FeLV tests) and general assessment questions. The surgical technician should do the recalls on any surgical case that they were a part of and did the release appointment for. The doctor may call back anybody that they like, but should definitely consider calling all new clients, major medical or surgical cases, and lab work that is not a simple positive/negative result. The receptionist would call any missed appointments.

Anyone can call vaccination and physical exam reminders that are overdue. Everybody or anybody can do the calls; you just need a script and some role playing at staff meetings. You might even consider hiring somebody just to do the callbacks—your "client communications specialist." Select the personnel to do the callbacks based upon what is correct for your practice, their telephone personality, and available personnel. Then decide when, how, and who! See Appendix 3 for additional ideas on who could do different callbacks. Don't let the job titles suggest that these are only for big practices. In a one-person practice the receptionist, tech, and assistant may all be the same person.

When to call? That depends upon the community that you live in. However, the greatest likelihood of catching somebody at home would be late afternoon. Try different times during the day. See what your success rate is. Don't forget the weekends!

The scripts should be simple and indicate concern. For example, "Mrs. Gerber, Dr. Cole and I were concerned about Baby's ears. How are they responding to the medication? Are you having any difficulties medicating the ears? Do you have any questions? Good, we look forward to seeing you again on the 27th for the recheck appointment." Each attempted and successful call needs to be documented and the results of the conversation or failure to get through placed in the medical record. Give at least three efforts at different times and on different days. After the third strike consider sending a letter such as the one in Appendix 3.

Reminders

As a part of Baby's visit she received her vaccinations, heartworm test, and a fecal assessment and went home with a bag of food. Each of these items may have a reminder linked to it. Whereas vaccinations will automatically generate a reminder for immunization review and annual life cycle consultation in a year, the fecal may be semi-annual or a dual spring and fall reminder. The heartworm test may generate a lab reminder for the annual test and a 6- or 9-month reminder for a medication refill. The food could be part of recall by the nutritional counselor and a reminder to pick up more food at the end of projected usage. Think of how impressed the client will be when they get a reminder that they should be just about finished with their bag of food and that you have one waiting for them.

Vaccinations are not the only reminder item. Most of us bought a computer to do all those mindless tasks that we humans constantly can't do right. The simplest was to be a cash drawer and keep the daily books. Most agree that the best moneymaker was a vaccine reminder. Since they come automatically tied to a vaccine, most of us get that one right. However the automatic reminder is normally the twelfth month. Do we really want to wait until the patient's protection has expired for the first reminder? We advocate sending the first reminder in the eleventh month. Forget the alphabet code; send a simple message that the client will understand. "Splash's protection against several infectious diseases will expire next month."

Progressive practices, seeing the controversial vaccine battle emerging, have already switched to a more important message. "Mia is due for her annual physical. Any protection she needs will also be discussed at that time." The second reminder is the traditional twelfth-month reminder. "Skeeter's protection is about to expire. Please make an appointment as soon as possible." The third reminder is most effective if it's a telephone call. "Dr. Weinstein and I are really worried that Cricket's protection has expired." For those not comfortable with this approach, the call may be, "The doctor and I missed Cricket this week. Is everything OK?" Or a letter may be sent instead of a postcard to draw attention to the importance of this event.

Numerous procedures that are done on a daily basis warrant a reminder or recall. Consider the following:

Thyroid levels: With initial prescription create a reminder for 4–6 weeks after starting for a "post pill test." Generate a reminder and recall that says, "Fluffy has been on her thyroid medication for 4–6 weeks now. She needs to have a follow-up assessment of her blood thyroid level so that we can make sure we are neither undercorrecting nor overcorrecting her level. This is a simple in-and-out visit. However, we need to collect the blood sample between four and six hours after she receives her morning pill. Once we establish her at a safe and therapeutic dosage, we will refill your prescription for one year prior to rechecking her and her thyroid level. Call today for an appointment."

Phenobarbital levels: As with the thyroid above, Phenobarbital is a drug that should be monitored routinely both for its therapeutic effects and its side effects. Based upon your comfort level, set up a program for a recall and reminder for phenobarbital levels and full laboratory profiles on a regular basis.

Glucose curves, digoxin, tapazole, potassium bromide, and any other drug requiring therapeutic monitoring can all generate automatic reminders either for refills or for lab assessment.

Repeat liver or kidney profiling, CBCs for autoimmune processes, and UAs for bladder stones can all generate reminders. Based upon your medical programs, set up reminders and recalls to bring people back in for their follow-up.

Postsurgical: Cruciate, MPL, FHO, TPO—when do you want to see them back?

Dentistry: Every exam should generate a dental reminder from one week to one year after the exam.

Heart murmurs: Repeat chest rads, ultrasounds, EKGs.

Spays and neuters: A novel concept—tie in a reminder to the first puppy vaccine to have a sterilization procedure done. Send a reminder or call at four months or older and encourage the procedure. You might even offer a population control discount to anyone responding to the reminder.

Allergens: When is it time for desensitization refills, medications, and hypoallergenic diets?

Anything and everything you do could fit into the reminder or recall category. So just do it!

In this one case, multiple forms of contact and communication were generated. What else can you develop recalls and reminders for? See Appendix 3 for more ideas. For virtually every physical assessment or diagnosis there should be a definitive period of time to schedule that recheck. You can develop a recheck protocol. It may read something like: Skin 14 days; Ears 10 days; Abscess—4d and 10 days. These are examples. Try to be uniform for each case and soon your front office will set up the recheck even before you turn in the travel sheet. You are limited only by your creativity. Here are a few ideas to get you started:

Recalls
- Any doctor exam
- Vaccinations
- Surgery
- Dentistry
- Medical procedures
- After lab test results
- After dispensing any of the new flea products

- Baths
- Boarding

Reminders
- Vaccinations
- Annual physicals
- Spay/ Neuter
- Medication testing and refills
- Retesting lab work
- Free tooth brushing lesson after dentistry
- Annual (or more frequent) dental reminder

Recheck Protocols

Ears, level I	14 days
Ears, level II	10 days
Ears, level III	7 days
Ears, level IV	3 days
Skin, level I	21 days
Skin, level II	14 days
Skin, level III	10 days
Skin, level IV	7 days
Dental disease, grade I	9–12 months
Dental disease, grade II	6 months
Dental disease, grade III	2 months
Dental disease, grade IV	2 weeks

Lab work:
  Therapeutic drug monitoring
  Chemical profiles for liver
  Chemical profiles for kidney
  Repeat urinalysis
Surgical rechecks

In Review

✓ Circle sheet has the 3 R's
  Recall ⌐
  Recheck ⊢ every pet gets one of these prior to departure!
  Remind ⌐

✓ Computer tracks and reminds you and your staff to do one of the above

✓ Recall by phone
✓ Recheck in person
✓ Remind by mail, fax, e-mail, or phone

No single program shows the client your caring attitude more than the 3 R's. It brings them back, it causes new client referrals, and it prevents things from getting lost in the shuffle. Most important, from a business standpoint, it makes the front door swing.

Client Retention

Have you ever looked at how much you spend each month on advertising or promotional efforts to lure new clients into your practice? Have you ever thought about giving that money to your staff? Why? Because they are the ones who can help guarantee the success of your practice by making certain that you retain each and every client who walks through the door or calls your practice.

For years, the Average Client Transaction has been the yardstick by which practices would compare themselves. This, however, is like the old myth: Is bigger really better?

Would you rather have 100 clients at $100 ACT? Or 200 clients at $60 ACT? What if those 100 clients only visited two times per year and the 200 clients visited four times per year? Which practice would you like?

100 clients × $100 × 2 = $20,000

200 clients × $60 × 4 = $48,000

Therefore, instead of looking at ACT, let's look at pets per household, number of pet visits per year, and annual revenue per pet or per client as a better measure of a practice's success. So, what is the trick to client retention and pet retention? A program designed to maintain contact with the client. A program designed to initiate contact if there is too long a period of time between contacts. A program designed to inquire about other pets in the household and to work to meet their needs.

These are the recovered client and recovered pet programs.

Recovered Pet Program—this means screening the existing clients entering the front door for other pets at home that have not been seen for the wellness programs at the practice. One of these "forgotten" animals is scheduled for an appointment each day, with a red "RP" placed in front of the name in the appointment log. Work out the numbers. ACT × 5 pets/week × 50 weeks a year × 3–6 visits per year per pet. A recovered pet per day with this program has an annual value of about $60,000 in increased annual income, mostly all net, because the overhead has already been paid. This program has many redundant features to ensure that at least one level catches that escaped pet. On the first phone call all pets should be viewed on the computer screen. The question should be asked whether we've forgotten anyone. When the client appears at the front desk, the same procedure should be repeated. The outpatient nurse reviews every pet's record as part of the intake or discharge program. Finally the doctor reviews every Patient Data Sheet (checkerboard square) in each pet's medical record as part of his or her history taking. Will all of these happen on every visit? Never. Hopefully at least one step will occur with each client visit.

Recovered Client Program—this is screening past clients who have not appeared for the recheck, have not returned for wellness care, have missed the second reminder card, or are a no-show for an appointment. One of these "forgotten" clients is scheduled for an appointment each day, with a red "RC" placed in front of the client's appointment on the log. Work out the numbers on a client's annual value (even at only 1.5 pets per household), and you will note that this program is about a $90,000 increase in annual income, mostly net, because the overhead has already been paid.

The secret is staff recognition during the RC and RP efforts. For the $150,000-plus additional income generated by the reception team's effort (RC = $90,000, RP = $60,000, therefore RC + RP = $150,000), the practice leadership can afford to be generous with pay raises and recognition monies.

Customer Service Is King

It may sound trite, it may sound trivial, but it works. People will pay more for service. The level of care and service that you provide will bond clients to you better than any coupon or giveaway that you have ever tried. People have come to recognize that service comes with a price. They will go for a discount on those commodity items where service is insignificant. However, if you provide value and service for the price that you charge, people will come back time and again.

How can we convert our practices into client advocates? Easily, by doing everything better than the way the human healthcare professionals do, as it pertains to client-centered services. Be available, be on time, be caring and compassionate, follow up and follow through, and provide full service in a single site. These are just a few concepts. However, it all starts with your paraprofessionals.

There are three people at minimum who communicate with the client before the doctor even sees the pet. These client contacts are points where you can win or lose clients. It may not make a difference how good you are as a schmoozer if your main receptionist is a loser. The client will talk to a receptionist on the phone, see a receptionist upon arrival, and be checked in by a technician. All this occurs before you get your 10 minutes of time. Anyone in the chain can be a weak link.

People-people are born not made. When you go through your hiring process, it is imperative to identify this trait. You can train anyone to answer the phone. You can't train everyone to answer the phone with a courteous smile on his or her face. You can train anyone to be an exam room tech. You can't train everyone to be a client and pet advocate, let alone emphasize and empathize. Caring and compassion have to ooze through the pores of a veterinary hospital staff. Therefore they must be empowered to make decisions that are in the best interests of the client, the pet, and the hospital without being required to get a supervisor's OK each time a question comes up.

Customer service is a skill. It is taking people-people and making them into yes-people. Teaching the art of thank-you's. Teaching the art of gentle persuasion. Teaching the art of offering multiple options to the clients that are also the options that are also best for the hospital. Client education is an imperative part of customer service. The more that is known about the medical condition being treated, the more information can be exchanged.

Training to Trust

To bring a practice into the next millennium will require staff training like never before offered. To be able to provide the care and service that our clients will demand, we must extend our use of all our paraprofessionals as members of our veterinary team. To be able to do this, we must train to trust. For our clients to trust our staff, we must trust our staff and their knowledge about what the practice needs and goals are. To be customer service advocates, we must define and redefine guidelines.

In school, they used to say, "See one, do one, teach one." Training a paraprofessional is not much different. Continuing education programs should be an integral part of an employee's performance planning. The information gathered at these programs should be returned to the practice. During staff meetings the employee should teach his or her cohorts lessons learned at CE. This teaching should then lead to the refining of a process and role playing until protocols are finally established, scripts are written, and programs are defined. These are documented either in writing or on videotape from which future employees are trained. They are also considered living documents and thus will change as the needs of the practice change.

For the 3 R's, the doctors and the paraprofessionals will define and assign which diseases will be rechecked and when. The vaccine series schedules, the splint or cast, or timing for suture or drain removal are defined by the doctors. The front office should recognize these and schedule accordingly. The circle sheet is used as the backup. The scripts, examples of which are in Appendix 4, should be personalized and modified for the comfort of the customer service advocate and the practice philosophy; however, the need of the pet is always emphasized.

When to do the callbacks, who should do them, and the script to use are individually defined.

Resources include Dale Carnegie, Telephone Co., Lisa Ford, and many more service-oriented courses.

Role playing is an excellent tool for staff meetings. There has to be some give and take. You must also define which recalls and client contacts you are willing to give up.

COMPUTER TRACKING AND PRODUCTION

✓ Travel sheet and 3 R's
✓ Doctor's responsibility
✓ Reminders linked to services, procedures, products, or pet's age
✓ Callback lists generated by computer
✓ Link client education handouts to travel sheet and to invoice codes

Tracking the success of various programs

Return rate per year
Average visits per year: National average
                                    Regional average
                                    Your average

Dollars spent per client per year: National average
                                    Regional average
                                    Your average

Longevity:
What percentage of your clients have not been seen within 12 months or 24 months?

Multiple pets:
What numbers of your households have multi-dog, multi-cat, multi-pet, or exotics?
Have you seen the other pet?

Turnover:
Reminders—percentage of reminders that come in off the first reminder, second reminder, third reminder
Rechecks—percentage of medical or surgical procedures that keep recheck appointments
Percentage of spay/neuter reminders that are seen
Percentage of dental reminders that are scheduled
Percentage of thyroid recheck reminders that are acted upon

The list goes on. Track trends for the above and any others. Note decreases and ascertain whether it is due to the receptionist, the timing of the reminder, or even the failure of the reminder to be sent.

The old Tom Cat axiom still stands. "If you don't measure it, it won't happen." If you measure the programs and develop the people to implement them, then the front door will swing.

The Appointment Book 2

The basis of making a successful appointment is offering the client two or three "yes" answers. The receptionist never says "No," but instead always offers positive alternatives. This doesn't mean that clients always get exactly what they request. They're just rarely told a flat "No!"

"The doctor can see you at 2 or 4 or tomorrow. Which do you prefer?"

"I want right now!!"

"The Doctor is in surgery, but you can drop Bud off now. He will be examined immediately by Sharon, our inpatient technician, and Doctor Talbot will see him as soon as surgery is finished or he can see you at 2 or 4." The receptionist must *smile* while talking to Mrs. Crotchety. Notice the word *no* was never used.

"Dr. Purcell is at a continuing education course this week to help her take better care of Spot. She can see you next Monday or Dr. Ross can see you today at 3 or tomorrow at 10. Which is better for you?"

It is always the client's choice. A key point is to train your receptionist to close the sale. Motivate the client or shopper to make an appointment. When Susan does our mystery shopping, she is always asked about the pet, but rarely asked to make an appointment.

My partner's final fallback for receptionists who can do nothing right no matter how hard they try is as follows:

"If none of these choices work for you, I'll have Dr. Gorrindo call you during his catch-up time at 3 p.m. today. Have a nice day!!"

Narratives

These are real names, procedures, and solutions in my practice. Use your own variations and the procedures already in place at your hospital. Make sure your receptionist knows your comfort level. When do you want to be interrupted for an emergency phone call or an irate client? Will you accept walk-ins? Should appointments always be taken before a walk-in, no matter how long they've waited? How long is too long? What should your receptionist say if an emergency is taken before an appointment? How should staff handle a new client with no money? Train the receptionist in these scenarios.

Better still, look at the examples in Appendix 4, then allow your team to develop their own narratives. In developing your own narratives, start by having the reception team compile a list of the most frequently asked questions or requested services. Make sure they have all the technical information necessary. Then let them develop narratives within their comfort zone following these guidelines:

> Relate to the client. Be empathetic to the client's concerns. Inform the client of the hospital's policy, procedure, or program. Be proud of the hospital's standard of care and explain it to the client. Whenever possible offer two "yes" answer choices in a closure question. Now offer two more "yes" options for appointments.

After the narrative is written, have them take turns saying it to each other. Role-play as client and receptionist. Change the wording until the receptionists are comfortable using it. By having the team develop their own narratives, they will buy in to the whole program.

After the narratives are developed and practiced, put them into effect. Then by all means, back up staff when they follow your policies. If you consistently override what the receptionist tells a client, you will train all your clients to talk only to you. Then you will spend your entire day on the phone earning receptionist wages rather than a doctor's salary. If this is already happening in your practice, reevaluate how you want to spend your time. Decide how you want your receptionist to handle recurring situations. Retrain your reception staff through role playing. Once they have the concept, let them do it. Trust them to handle these situations, back their decisions, and go back to being a doctor.

In-House Appointments

Step two is the in-house appointment. This is the recheck from the 3 R's in Chapter One. Make that next appointment before Mrs. Donahue leaves the office. Otherwise she'll forget and so will you. Make the appointment and give her a calendar sticker, recheck refrigerator card, or whatever take-home reminder fits your style. Call her if she misses the appointment. What if she just doesn't know her schedule? Use another "yes" answer.

"I'll make myself a note to call you (recall) in a few days. Is home or office better?" *Smile.* Two or three days later call Mrs. Donahue and remind her that Dr. Ross wanted to see Charity back next week. Does she know her schedule yet?

High-Density Scheduling

If I told you high-density scheduling in your appointment book could increase your volume by 30 to 40 percent, would you be interested? All of the following elements are necessary for this to happen. There certainly are many variations, but the key elements are essential—use of staff extenders, scheduling rooms not doctors, 10-minute blocks, and day admittance for workups.

The use of various staff extenders in your practice is covered in Chapters Three and Four. You may use any or all of them to extend your availability to your clients and patients. Briefly, an outpatient nurse does wellness exams, medication dispensing, and discharge instructions while you're in the next room. Backroom technicians have assistants, and this team does all the workups, IVs, anesthesia, x-rays, blood draws, and preps—everything except diagnoses and surgery. This frees you to have high-quality, low-quantity time with your patients and clients. The use of these extenders to do "nondoctor" functions such as client education, technical skills, and paperwork allows you to see 30 to 40 percent more appointments in the same amount of time. This will not only increase your gross and net, but also provide your clients with greater access time. For those practices on the borderline of needing another doctor, it makes a big difference between a high-net, one-doctor practice and a low-net, two-doctor practice. Except for those single-doctor practices taking their own emergency calls, it almost always makes more sense to hire another tech or assistant before another doctor.

Who determines the number of blocks it takes a given doctor to see a given problem? The doctor knows best! Right? Wrong! Bite your tongue, swallow your pride, and let your experienced receptionist handle the appointment book. Without your knowledge, Carrie already schedules differently for her five doctors. If you ask her, and she's not afraid of lightening bolts, she'll tell you. She knows better than you do how long each doctor takes for various problems. She even knows to add an extra 10 minutes for your mother-in-law. The doctors should set some basic starting points for various types of appointments. They're then defined and discussed at a meeting with the reception team. Next the receptionists implement them. The basic starting point is a 20-minute appointment in two 10-minute blocks. Add 10 minutes for a new graduate, an extra patient, a new puppy for first vaccines, a geriatric workup, or a severe dermatology or medical case. Only schedule 10 minutes for a quick recheck, drain removal, or suture removal. Build from there depending on your practice's personal preferences.

Let the reception team play with the variables and each doctor's style. In 90 days re-evaluate. Until then, leave the team alone! Have everyone write down both good and bad points of the new system to discuss in 90 days, but don't nag them on a daily basis. After 90 days schedule another meeting. Honestly, how's it going? If the doctor is standing around, you can shorten some blocks. If the doctor is always behind, it stimulates a lot of questions. Do you think you're faster than you are? Do you fully utilize your outpatient nurse? Should you do more day admits? Are the times you've set just unrealistic? Should you have technician appointments for suture and drain removals? Should you schedule your assistants differently or have one per room instead of one per doctor?

Schedule two rooms in 10-minute blocks, staggered. There are sample appointment pages in Vol. 2, and several vendors now have copies of this type of appointment book that even show catch-up time already shaded in. Some computer schedulers are already set up for this system. See Figure 2.1 for the rest of this discussion. Remember, 10 minutes is allowed for suture removal (possibly by a technician), drain removal, or quick rechecks. Twenty minutes is for routine appointments. You get an extra 10 for an extra animal, new puppy—first visit, severe geriatric, or medical problem. Let your reception team decide. Try to alternate difficult appointments between the two columns. Don't book back-to-back new puppies or severe problems. Alternate with rechecks or second vaccinations. This is done in Exam Room 2 in Figure 2.1 for the first half of the afternoon. Why did the receptionist mark off 2:15 in Room 2? This is in order to start off the staggering of the two rooms. The same thing occurs at 3:55 after the catch-up time. What are all the Xs? This is how Carrie marks off the extra 10-minute blocks needed in one room for the type of appointment and the matching blocks in the next room to keep appointments staggered. How can Dr. Haig be in with Sue Siple and George Halyak at the same time? He's not! As discussed below, the outpatient nurse is either doing the initial TPR (temperature, pulse, and respiration) on Midge in the first five minutes in Room 2 or the discharge on Duz in the last five minutes of Room 1.

Once the reception team is trained, the appointment book is a "no-touch zone" for doctors. Stay out of it! Book at least one catch-up time in the morning and one in the afternoon. Use 10 to 30 minutes across both columns; you decide how much time your practice requires. In this

APPOINTMENT LOG SAMPLE

	DR. H. EXAM ROOM 1					DR. HAIG EXAM ROOM 2			
	Client's Name	Pet's Name	Client Concern	Phone		Client's Name	Pet's Name	Client's Concern	Phone
2:15	Halyak	Duz	Ears	****	2:15	XXXXX	XXXX	XXXX	XXX
2:25	XXXXX	XXX	XXX	XXX	2:25	Siple	Midge	Drain tube	****
2:35	Rivera	2 new	Puppy		2:35	Xxxxxxx	Xxxxxx	Xxxxxxx	Xxxxx
2:45		Puppies	Plan		2:45	Xxxxxxx	Xxxxxx	Xxxxxxx	Xxxx
2:55	Xxxxxxxx	xxxx	Xxxxxx	Xxxxx	2:55	Duzan	Snicker	2nd Pup P	****
3:05	Truax	Fred	Geriatric	*****	3:05	Xxxxx	Xxxxx	Xxxxx	Xxxx
3:15	Xxxxxxxx	Xxxx	Physical	Xxxx	3:15	XXXX	XXXX	XXXXX	XXXX
3:25	XXXXXX	XXXX	XXXX	XXX	3:25	Xxxxxx	Xxxxxx	Xxxxxxxx	xxxxx
3:35	Catch-up	Time	Catch-up	Time	3:35	Catch-up	Time	Catch-up	Time
3:45					3:45				
3:55	Catanzaro	Max	Abscess	9800	3:55	XXXXX	XXXX	XXXX	XXX
4:05	XXXXX	XXXX	XXXX	XXX	4:05	Strattmn	Queen	Heart	6996
4:15	XXXXXX	XXXX	XXXXX	XXX	4:15	XXX	XXX	Murmur	XXX
4:25	Leake	Ralph	Rechk	0754	4:25	XXXX	XXXX	XXXX	XXX
4:35	Xxxxx	Xxxx	Ear SX	Xxx	4:35	Howell	Nikki	Eye Exam	3693
4:45	XXXX	XXX	XXXX	XXX	4:45	XXXX	XXX	XXX	XXX
4:55	Seibert	New	Kitten	1925	4:55	XXXX	XXX	XXXX	XXX
5:05	XXXX	Kitten	Plan	XXX	5:05	XXXXX	XXXX	XXXXX	XXX
5:15	Catch-up	Time	Catch-up	Time	5:15	Catch-up	Time	Catch-up	Time
5:25	Catch-up	Time	Catch-up	Time	5:25	Catch-up	Time	Catch-up	Time
5:35					5:35				
5:45					5:45				
5:55					5:55				
6:05					6:05				
6:15					6:15				
6:25					6:25				
6:35					6:35				
6:45					6:45				
6:55					6:55				

FIGURE 2.1

case, Dr. Haig is a new graduate, so we gave him two catch-up times. If you're on schedule, these times are for callbacks, checking lab work, and x-rays. If you're way behind, these times literally catch you up.

There are several options in scheduling to fit your practice. The morning outpatient doctor can rotate to inpatient in the afternoon. This allows him or her to evaluate the morning workups, do minor procedures or even rotate into surgery. Some practices even have an inpatient doctor who accepts cases all day long from the outpatient doctors, while the outpatient doctor continues to see appointments. This really requires confidence in your associates and good medical records. Another option is to schedule one-hour staggered lunches for procedures and review of cases. If you have no surgery or major workups, you get a real chance to sit down and eat.

In practices with an inpatient doctor, he or she sees all walk-ins and emergencies. This keeps the outpatient doctors on schedule and ensures that the regularly scheduled appointments aren't rushed. Schedule a telephone time in late morning and another just before rush hour in the afternoon or evening. This really should be in addition to catch-up time. If we use Dr. Gorrindo's plan for recalls during telephone time, this "guarantees" the receptionist a time when you will contact the cranky client. If you get in the habit of telling your clients about this when they leave their pet, it also makes your day easier and decreases telephone traffic drastically for the front desk. Tell your client you will call them at an approximate time. This time corresponds to your telephone time as well as to the normal time lab results are received. Hopefully the receptionist doesn't get multiple phone calls checking to see if Buffy's lab work or x-rays are done. Once your receptionist trusts you, Mrs. Mack will be asked on the first unscheduled call if you have already promised a time to call her with results. After an affirmative answer, she will then be asked politely to wait until then for your call.

In a standard 20-minute appointment, the first five minutes is for a quick wellness exam, additional history, and TPR by the outpatient nurse. The doctor comes in, does a more through physical (doesn't have to do TPR), and addresses client concerns and problems noted by the OPN. Then s/he makes a tentative diagnosis and diagnostic or treatment plan. At this point a decision is made to either do a day admit (see Chapter Four) or dispense and go home. See Chapter Three for more details on how to use the OPN effectively. The OPN then returns and either dispenses medications with instructions and client education or admits to the back room for diagnostics and treatment or quick blood draw and necessary injections.

Whichever occurs, that exam room is empty in 20 minutes for the next patient. In a perfect traffic flow and schedule the client has 20 minutes of quality time. This was identified in the Pfizer study as the maximum tolerance level, no matter how much you think clients love you. Has anyone seen the key yet? Twenty minutes of quality time including discharge instructions are better than most of us have time to deliver, but the doctor only spent 10 minutes in the room! By using staff for everything except medicine and surgery, the doctor gives the client excellent care, caring discharge instructions, and handouts in half the time. No hurried "Here's your pills, read the label" at our hospitals. There's even a caring staff member before and after each visit for the clients to ask those questions they were afraid to ask the doctor!

The next mind leap is to book rooms not doctors. Whether you're using an appointment book or a computer screen, you need, physically and on the page, two exam rooms for each doctor seeing appointments. You don't have that many exam rooms? I'll bet if you schedule one doctor as surgery/inpatient, or in bigger practices, one as surgery and one as inpatient, you just "found" extra exam rooms. Even if there are only two doctors, one can be doing surgery while the other sees appointments. Without "squeezing procedures between appointments" you'll both be more efficient.

In a one-doctor practice the same principles apply. The OPN in the morning, becomes the surgery tech midday. With high-density scheduling of surgery and appointments, as well as proper staff utilization, one doctor can produce 40 percent more. You then use the above methods to stagger appointments with your two or three "yes" answers. Never book two new puppies or serious geriatrics in adjoining rooms. Squeeze a suture removal or recheck ears in between those types of appointments. Role-play appointments at a staff meeting with the receptionist both "on the telephone" and in the appointment book. The first time you try the high-density scheduling, only book a morning or afternoon's worth of appointments. Then schedule a meeting to review the results. Be open and honest, not belittling and with no finger-pointing. Then try a whole day or a Saturday. Review again!

Even though I said try it for 90 days, that doesn't mean without feedback. Schedule a brief 20-minute meeting over coffee for feedback. Never discuss the situation in front of a client, especially when you're feeling frustrated. Listen to the staff's ideas and concerns about improving the program. If confusion reigns, regroup and retry. It is really awkward for everyone to get used to at first. This is a total change in habits for everyone. Imagine no client waiting, 40 percent more "yes" answers for appointments, and you guessed it, more money for staff bonuses! It's really worth all the hassle to break those old habits. (OK, for Tom Cat, I'll call them paradigms.) It takes a lot of training for you, your staff, and your clients. Example:

> "Mrs. Chichester, I'm going to have Denise call you in a few days to see how Toby is doing. Then we'll schedule an appointment with Sandy to take out those sutures. If you have any problems in between you call either one of them or me."

See how you subtly retrain the client and do an in-house referral of the next appointment to your staff? The same technique can be used to introduce a new associate or to get set up for your vacation by referring to the relief veterinarian.

As discussed previously, you must define the outpatient nurse's exam and history-taking responsibility within your practice. This should compliment your own exam and history, not duplicate it. For example, teach your OPN to explain that the stethoscope is being used to take a pulse, not evaluate heart sounds. Otherwise some clients will ask why you both had to listen to the heart. Both the receptionist and OPN should write down any client concerns followed by a box indicating an action needed on your part. Often they will be told things the client forgets to tell the doc. I don't think it's productive to have you both take an exhaustive history. My OPN does a TPR, diet, any other complaints, and an outta-there type exam. In areas with heartworm prevalence, the OPN can effectively begin the conversion to an annual physical program. Prior to the doctor's entrance, fecal and blood samples can be obtained as part of the annual physical. An interesting addition to this program is baseline blood screens. Again, your practice must define these parameters. IDEXX Laboratories, Inc. has a good starting point for various age groups. You must modify them for your geographical area and comfort zone. The OPN then explains that you recommend XYZ as a baseline for this age group and that it can be done at the same time, since blood is being drawn anyway. This will serve as a baseline as well as preanesthetic blood work for any procedures that need to be done in the next 3 to 6 months. Feline leukemia and immunodeficiency virus testing may be handled in a similar fashion.

If a caring receptionist has the proper tools in the computer, annual post pill T4, potassium bromide, or Phenobarbital blood levels may be scheduled at the proper time of day to coincide with the annual exam. If these databases are standard in your practice, part of your technician and receptionist's training includes scheduling all these automatically at the time of appointment. The real beauty of this system is that all this scheduling, sampling, and testing is done without any participation on your part after the initial client training. The ultimate example of this system occurred while I was on site at Carriage Hills Animal Hospital. I walked into the exam room with the doctor. Michelle turned to us and said, "Fluffy has had blood drawn for her heartworm test and geriatric physical. We also have a fecal sample. She will be spending the day for the rest of her tests. She's also decided to spend the night at our resort. If the tests are all satisfactory, she will have her teeth cleaned tomorrow." The doctor and I should have just turned around and walked out! Seriously, he completed the physical exam, had no further recommendations, said "Thank-you," and went on to the next exam. How long would all of that taken in your practice? The doctor's actual time in the exam room was less than 10 minutes, and most of that was socializing!

Consultation versus Examination

For years we have called the doctor's patient diagnostic exam and client consultation, the sharing of knowledge and skills, by one term: *examination*. In fact, if you're old enough, it was first called an *office call*. We were comfortable with this misnomer, even to the extent of hiding the professional effort inside a "vaccination fee," that is until the superstore down the street said that an exam was included with all vaccinations. Panic was a common response, but clarity in services rendered and itemized listing within the practice billing was not.

Then the retrospective vaccine panic hit the profession. Some people believed that the vaccinations were dangerous, and in pursuit of research dollars they published antidotal information not substantiated by the traditionally severe drug evaluation criteria. Again, panic was a common response, but clarity in services rendered and itemized listing within the practice billing was not. However, this time more practices started looking for an alternative to burying everything inside the vaccination fee.

The clarity of practice billing was not the goal, just what they could advertise to beat the competition and media blitz. Please stop the insanity. Look at what your practice is doing and start quantifying what your quality of care stands for in the community. Look at a current application of reality and truth in performance:

An animal deserves an annual life cycle consultation with the doctor. (One dog year is equal to about seven people years, and that is long enough for any living entity to wait for a wellness evaluation!)

A nurse's wellness examination is done at every entry into the hospital, but the doctor's diagnostic examination is done only when the pet is sick or with the annual life cycle consultation. This is a critical step in maintaining the pet in a well state, due to the other factors that will be discussed even when the pet appears healthy (as discussed below).

The consultation will offer discussions about the immunization and protection programs available, as well as when the pet needs to access those services. It will likely be at a time separate from the consultation, so the cost of the annual life cycle consultation will seldom be additive, unless the client requests that immediate care be rendered.

Screening programs for better breath (dentistry), internal body system changes (blood chemistry), and even surveillance of the aging process (radiology and electrocardiograms) will be discussed and scheduled on an as-needed basis.

Families that hike with their pet, take them on vacation, or just live near the fields and woods may need additional protection; that is also discussed and planned during the doctor's consultation.

Fleas and ticks, as well as some internal parasites, can be deterred from attacking the pet. These alternatives will be discussed during the consultation, and options will be provided for the client's consideration.

As you can see, most of the consultation elements above require: 1) participative listening; 2) assessment of internal, external, or environmental dangers; and 3) subsequent client communications. If your practice takes the time to listen to clients, healthcare access is increased in most A and B clients, and often even in the C clients. If the practice tries to do all of the above with only doctors, you cannot afford the effort. If you use an outpatient nursing program concurrent with high-density scheduling, as discussed in Vol. 2, the clients will begin to equate veterinary healthcare with other healthcare delivery models. Human outpatient clinics use three to five examination rooms per doctor and dentists use four to eight chairs per doctor. Clients will start to understand that technicians are really nurses with exceptional skills and knowledge about companion animals and, generally, with far better abilities and capabilities than most of their human medicine counterparts.

So, undifferentiated examination by habit or clarity in quality with the consultation—the choice is yours today. With failure to change, you will either lose the option or become an "old timer"; neither role will attract the quality client to your practice. Slow death is painful . . . and for the want of a horseshoe nail, the war was lost!

Teamwork between Exam Rooms

This is the overlap area that feeds into Chapter Four. There are many variations. Assume that you are using the basic high-density schedule of two rooms and one outpatient nurse per doctor. Who fills the prescriptions? Who loads the rooms? Who takes the animals to the back?

There are many variations. Here are a few:

The OPN fills the Rx's, takes them back into the exam room, and explains them to the client. In this variation, a receptionist does checkout at the front desk. Either a receptionist or OPN may load the exam room.

In the second variation a receptionist position is created that is called a floater. This person loads rooms, fills scripts, and runs laps all day!

A great variation for traffic flow, especially if you have a back hallway with an outside exit, is exam room checkout. With this method you probably need two OPNs. The OPN fills the meds, prints out the receipt in the pharmacy or exam room, and charges the client right there. The client and patient exit the side door and never go up front again.

If you are doing a day admit as discussed in Chapter Four, either the OPN or the doctor may take a patient to the back for diagnostics or treatment. The patient is then turned over to the inpatient team. More variations of this procedure are given in Chapter Four.

Training to Trust

As discussed at every turn in these chapters and many of the other ISUP texts, training the staff is the key to successful use of veterinary extenders. Staff training times are essential. Use role playing to increase the confidence of the reception team with their narratives. Have the doctors play their worst cranky clients to allow OPNs to develop the proper skills to handle clients alone in the exam rooms. They too need narratives to use for recommended testing procedures, day admits, go home instructions, and any other routine communications with clients.

Computer Appointment Books

Several computer vendors currently have on-line appointment books that are adaptable to high-density scheduling. Some you have to fake out. Give the doctor two numbers or two names. Doctor S and Doctor Smith become rooms one and two as in Figure 2.1. To move the telephone receptionist off the front desk and into a separate room requires an on-line appointment book. This removes stress from the front desk. The client no longer perceives rudeness when ignored to answer the phone. It also allows peace and quiet for the receptionist answering the phone. With computerized appointment books, tracking the appointment fill rate, the number of no-shows, and the number of unfilled appointments is no longer so labor intensive. Whether done manually or by computer, tracking these numbers is an effective way to monitor efficiency and rate of front door swing. Progressive measures include searching the computer database for various ratios:

✓ Number of dentals per office call
✓ Number of annual life cycle consultations per vaccine or patient
✓ Number of dentals per doctor
✓ Number of missed rechecks: Per recheck
                               Per doctor
                               Per client(s)

Effective use of the appointment book, high-density scheduling, and narrative training of the receptionists will go a long way toward making the front door swing as needed, discussed in Chapter One. The appointment book in many ways is the brain of the practice just like the treatment room is its heart!

Outpatient Programs and Procedures

3

Veterinary medicine has become a competitive world where you must find ways to differentiate yourself from your colleagues. The best place to do this is in the level of client service your practice provides. Remember, there may be three or more paraprofessional contacts with a client before a doctor sees the patient:

- The phone or walk-in contact with the receptionist
- The arrival for the appointment greeting
- The outpatient technician

How was the telephone handled? Was the client greeted expeditiously and with a smile? Did the technician handle the client and patient gently? All of these exposures occur before the doctor even enters the picture. This is why client service is king!

Besides making client service a priority, what other things can be done to create a feeling of patient advocacy? Following are some programs discussed in Chapter One that can be developed to reward, encourage, and bond clients to your practice.

Preferred Client Programs

Once you have an established relationship, you want to keep that relationship. One way to do this is to appeal to a universal desire to have choices or options. A preferred client program rewards established clients with choices for their veterinary care.

An established or preferred client may be defined as:

one who has had a complete physical examination and consultation by
    a doctor within a 12-month period;
one who has maintained all wellness parameters up to date; or
one who has the need for follow-up care.

What are wellness parameters? These are the minimum standards of
care for a particular species based on your region of the country or
your personal belief. They are the components of the checkerboard
square called the Patient Data Sheet (Volume 2) in the medical record
system. These are items that every pet should be screened for by the receptionist, the outpatient nurse, and finally the doctor. What are these
parameters in your practice?
They may include:

DOGS	CATS
DHPPC	FVRCCP
Bordetella	FeLV
Rabies	Rabies
Lyme	FIP
Fecal	Fecal
Heartworm	FeLV Skin /FIV Test
Dental Grade	Dental Grade
Diet	Diet

These are just a few of the most common items that may make up
the wellness parameters. Not all are applicable to every practice. If you
don't use it in your practice, don't put it on your form. If it's on your
form, require that it be screened on every visit. Screening may be as
simple as verifying that the vaccine box is filled in and the dates are
current.

A client who meets the specifically defined standards for your practice becomes eligible for various options for their pet's healthcare
needs.

1. Tech examinations and vaccinations (if legal in your state)
2. Doctor wellness exam and vaccinations
3. Free dental grading and examinations
4. Preferred availability for boarding and bathing
5. Any other parameters or services you want to provide

Dental Care Programs

It's time to reward clients for proactive dental care. We have been in the rut of charging similarly for all levels of dental care. The two-year-old golden retriever with slight dental calculus and the 12-year-old Yorkie with pus-mouth have been charged the same for cleaning, polishing, fluoride, anesthetic, etc. Why? Just because. ... It's easier not to think about changing.

Consider that dental care is a labor-intensive procedure. The two-year-old golden is a 20-minute procedure; the Yorkie a 55-minute procedure. But you charge the same. Consider creating four levels of dental care with a differential fee schedule for the four levels. Using the picture on the CET Handout ("Pets Have Teeth, Too") or any other brochure, create your own demonstrable and measurable guidelines. These are your four grades of dental disease and act as the starting point for your dental care program.

Next, insist that every mouth entering the hospital attached to a pet (except for the odd blue-tongued dogs) have a dental grade assigned to it. The entire paraprofessional staff should be trained to flip a lip to grade the level of dental disease. The grade is entered into the medical record, noted on the circle sheet, and thus linked to a reminder as discussed earlier.

The grading of teeth provides for the following:

1. a means of creating a pricing differential for the different levels of dental disease,
2. a means of rewarding those who make the effort to maintain their pet's teeth,
3. a means of creating a computer tracking system to enhance client communication, and
4. a means of linking staff to promoting proactive dental care.

Chapter Four also outlines the creation of dental care inpatient teams and details staff training on the importance of dental care. Examples of differential pricing and what each includes are in Appendix 1.

Life Cycle Programs

Geriatric programs/golden year programs/senior programs—not anymore. There have been numerous efforts to create different variations on this theme. Packages or programs that include everything from blood tests to radiology to ultrasound have been put together. To make these programs work you cannot start them at age eight or nine or some other randomly chosen age. The program must be a part of a lifelong wellness program.

So instead of providing a senior citizen special, look at life cycle programs. These could include:

Puppy/kitten programs
Teenage programs
Gen-X programs
Middle age programs
Maintenance programs
Progressive programs
Mellowing programs
Any other you can identify

Call them what you want. Set the age breaks wherever you want. But create levels of care that encourage ongoing preventative and screening tests for healthy pets at different stages of their lives.

The goal within any program is to bond the client and pet to your practice and to provide them with more services at a more affordable price, or bang for the buck. Life cycle programs are developed to provide wellness or preventative care at the various stages of a pet's life.

You can set the program up to cover any stages. Food companies have used the stages of puppy, maintenance, and senior. People are considered neonate, infant, pediatric, teen, generation X, middle age, geriatric, CTD (circling the drain), or buried. I would encourage using three or four categories. Consider the following:

Kitten/Puppy (Pediatric): Birth to one year
Young Adult: One year to five years
Middle age Adult: six years to eight years
Older Adult: Nine years and above

These are wellness and preventative programs, so for each category you should set your wellness parameters. Create an inclusive package with all parameters that you want to monitor. Identify your actual fee for *all* the services if provided at the same time. Provide an incentive (discount, giveaway, etc.) to encourage follow-through with the package.

At each stage of development you should be preparing the client for the next stage. Try to develop scripts, e.g., "We will monitor blood samples annually to identify changes before they become a problem. As your pet gets older, we will be testing more and more parameters so as not to miss anything." These statements help your paraprofessionals present things in the same fashion.

Examples of wellness/preventative/life cycle packages are in Appendix 1. Figure 3.1 is an example of wellness programs available in my practice for pets older than nine years. As you can see, there are three different levels of care, with room for additional options.

Customize the package to your specific philosophy, specific demographic location, and client base. The ultimate goal is to prepare the client each year for the subsequent year's events. Appendix 1 starts this process with puppies and works up to older adults (Figure 3.1). Hopefully, clients start coming in and saying, "Hi, I'm here for Hope's annual life cycle assessment. Here are her urine and fecal samples. Can we also update her vaccinations while you are drawing her blood sample?"

Dermatological Based Programs—Skin, Ears, Fleas, Etc.

In Southern California, 60 percent of the medical consultations that we have are ear or skin related. With the advent of the high-tech flea control products, we are seeing the true cases of atopy, food allergies, or scabies and their associated pruritus. The need for frequent reassessments to monitor responses to therapy is frustrating for both the client and the veterinary practice. The client's usual response is either to ask, "Do I have to pay for all their rechecks?" or a no-show.

Skin

As practitioners, we tend to assume a diagnosis with an itchy dog by inspection and experience. However, not every itchy dog is itchy for the same reason. You would be surprised at the willingness of clients to rule out certain things to help identify a cause rather than just reaching for the steroids, itch shot, or cortisone.

So let's put together a skin package. A thorough skin workup may include any or all of the following or more:

- Physical exam and consultation
- Skin scrape for mites

Program for: OLDER ADULT (>9 YEARS)

ITEM	REG. CHG	LEVEL 1	LEVEL 2	LEVEL 3	OPTIONS
PE/Consult		•	•	•	
FVRCP DHPPC		•	•	•	
FeLV Bordetella		•	•	•	
FIP Lyme		•	•	•	
Rabies		• If needed	• If needed	• If needed	
FeLV/FIV test Heartworm test		•	•	•	
Fecal		•	•	•	
Deworm		•	•	•	
Rx program Rx sentinel		•	•	•	
Weight		•	•	•	
Screening blood test		12 tests	Thyroid	12 tests Thyroid	
Urinalysis		•	•	•	
Ld. II EKG		•	•	6 lead	
Hip/back rads					•
Chest rads				•	
Tear test		•	•	•	
Glaucoma (IOP) screen		•	•	•	
Dental disease screen		•	•	•	
DISCOUNT					
FREE GOODS					
COST TO CLIENT					

FIGURE 3.1

- Skin smear for yeast, bacteria, etc.
- Fungal culture-DTM
- Biopsy
- Skin culture and sensitivity
- Allergy testing
- Thyroid and other endocrine tests
- Recheck
- Refill
- Recheck
- Refill
- ad infinitum

Many clients would like to be able to budget for their chronically itchy pet's skin care. Of course, there are others who just come in for a shot for their pet's itch. Again, you could create three levels of skin care packages. Prepaid packages or monthly withdrawal packages allow clients to budget, and they receive a break for going for the package.

By providing the rechecks for free (at least in their eyes), you should get greater compliance and more follow-ups to monitor the cases. For the client to appreciate these packages they need to see or perceive savings. It's the rechecks and refills that they get peeved about, so encourage these within the discount built into the package. See Figure 3.2 for an example of skin care package pricing.

Ears

Just as in skin care, ear care frustrations come from failure to follow up and the hesitancy for a good thorough ear flush under sedation. Clients just want the Band-Aid approach to ear problems. Encourage the rechecks, ear flushes, and follow-throughs by creating a package (see Figure 3.3). You could even offer a discount on a lateral ear or total ear ablation surgery for any client who has gone through one of the packages above.

Think about it; you could create your own package for any common problem that you see on a daily basis. Again the goal is to provide bang for the buck, ensure the perception of increased care and value, and bond the client to your practice. Here are some other recurring problems to consider for packages:

Program for: SKIN DISEASES

ITEM	REG. CHG	LEVEL 1	LEVEL 2	LEVEL 3	LEVEL 4
PE/Consult		•	•	•	•
Skin scrape		•	•	•	•
Skin cytology			•	•	•
Fungal culture		•	•	•	•
Injection		•	•	•	•
Injection			• (e.g. IVM)	•	•
Oral Rx		•	•	•	•
Oral Rx		•	•	•	•
Topical			•	•	•
Shampoo		•	•	•	•
Flea control—oral/injectable		•	10% off	10 % off	15% off
Flea control—topical		•	10% off	10 % off	15% off
Diet supplement			•	•	•
Sedate				•	•
Biopsy				•	•
Skin C & S				•	•
Allergy test					•
Antigens					•
Blood profile				•	•
Thryoid profile					•
Adrenal profile					option
Rechecks		2 free	4 free	6 free	8 free
DISCOUNT					
FREE GOODS					
COST TO CLIENT					

FIGURE 3.2

Program for: EAR DISEASES

ITEM	REG. CHG	LEVEL 1	LEVEL 2	LEVEL 3	LEVEL 4
PE/Consult		•	•	•	•
Skin scrape			•	•	•
Ear cytology		•	•	•	•
Fungal culture			•	•	•
Injection		•	•	•	•
Injection			• (e.g. IVM)	•	•
Oral Rx		•	•	•	•
Oral Rx			•	•	•
Topical		•	•	•	•
Topical			•	•	•
Ear cleaning		•	•	•	•
Flea control—oral/injectable			10% off	10 % off	15% off
Flea control—topical			10% off	10 % off	15% off
Diet supplement			•	•	•
Sedate				•	•
Ear flush				•	•
Ear C & S				•	•
Allergy test					•
Antigens					•
Blood profile				•	•
Thryoid profile					•
Adrenal profile					option
Rechecks		2 free	4 free	6 free	8 free
Repeat ear cytology		2 free	4 free	6 free	8 free
Rx refills		10% off	12 % off	15% off	15% off
Sedate and flush			Inc. 2	Inc. 3	Inc. 4
Lateral ear Sx					$200 off
DISCOUNT					
FREE GOODS					
COST TO CLIENT					

FIGURE 3.3

KCS-keratoconjunctivitis sicca (consider early age screening as part
    of your life cycle packages for predisposed breeds)
Glaucoma (same here for early age screening)
Heart murmurs with and without congestive heart failure
Chronic renal failure
Corneal ulcers
Chemotherapy
Bladder stones

For any package you put together you need the following:

1. buy-in and compliance by all doctors,
2. buy-in and compliance by all staff,
3. good client educational and marketing tools, and
4. a complete and thorough understanding of the disease process

Drug Monitoring Programs

Another common source for failed follow-through is with the use of
drugs on a long-term basis. Examples include: thyroid supplements,
antithyroid medications, phenobarbital, potassium bromide, and even
heartworm preventative.

Convince the client of the importance of follow-up when the medications are initially prescribed. Accomplish the follow-up with programs or packages and use your value-added software to generate reminders.

The packages should include refills, retests, recheck consultations,
and screening blood samples for drug side effects where appropriate.
For example:

Thyroid	Phenobarbital	Tapazole
Initial Rx	Initial Rx	Initial Rx
Recheck T4	Recheck Pheno	Recheck T4
at 1 mo	level at 1 mo	and CBC 1 mo
Refills	Refills	Refill
Recheck T4	Recheck Pheno	Recheck T4
at 1 year	at 6 mo	& CBC q 1 mo
Refills	Refills	Refills
Recheck T4	Recheck Pheno	Recheck T4 and
annually	and liver	CBC q 6 mo
Profile annually	Profile q 6 mo	

Again, these are only guidelines and may not either be complete enough for your practice or be too often for your philosophy.

Frequent Visit Programs

A mainstay of the American economy has become the frequent buyer/flyer program. Clients are constantly coming in and saying, "It seems like I'm here every day." Well, if they really and truly are, and they are bonded to you, why not reward them for their persistence?

✓ Frequent Bath Cards
   After X baths get 1 free.
✓ Frequent Boarder Cards
   Board X nights get (1) free bath; or (2) free nights; or (3) free exam; or you decide.
✓ Frequent Food Purchases
   Buy __ bags/cases get the next one free.
   (The food companies love these and will often reimburse you for the free bag.)

The ultimate goal as outlined earlier—repeat business! Then blow their socks off with client service!

Monitoring Programs from an Outpatient Basis

All these programs are great on paper. However, they must be put into place and utilized. They must be monitored and tracked. They must be modified to meet changing technology and changing client demands.

Ideas on Monitoring

Volume 2 (page 341) contains a chart listing various procedures with a month-by-month monitor. This is one way to track services provided. The chart should be personalized for your practice and your practice philosophy. For example, not everybody does ACL surgeries. However, you might monitor ACL surgery referrals or diagnoses.

Other ways to monitor programs are ratios. Of all the new puppy or kitten exams that you do, how many clients invest in the program? Of all the skin exams that you do, how many invest in each level of skin care? What is your return on your dental reminders?

Here are some others to consider:

New kitten: FeLV tests to new kitten exams
Recommend: 1:1 ratio.

New puppy/kitten: intestinal parasite exams to new kitten and new puppy exams
Recommend: 1:1 ratio.
Ever heard of a fecal loop? (Don't do this in front of the client. They see how far you go in and think you're cleaning their ears!)

New kitten/puppy packages sold: new kittens/puppies seen to packages sold
Optimal 1:1 ratio; Realistic 1:8 ratio. Same for new puppies.

Baseline lab work to annual physical examinations
As more packages are sold, should get closer to 1:1; more realistically 1:8.

Heartworm tests to annual canine physical exams
Depends upon personal and demographic needs. In the Southeast should be 1:1. In Orange County, California, it may be closer to 1:10. Also, this may vary depending on whether you are testing annually or less frequently.

Vaccine titers (a new concept)

Parvo + distemper titers: Parvo-distemper vaccinations

Quite controversial—do titers define protection? Can we safely vaccinate less frequently? This is still to be determined.

Geriatric profiles: geriatric exams

Optimally: 1:1 ratio; Realistically: 1:10 ratio.

Six-month-old dogs and cats: six-month-old dogs and cats spayed or neutered

Track this using your $20k reminder machine.

Start to Use Your Computer to Market Your Practice

Breed prevalence for certain diseases is well documented—thyroid disease in cockers, goldens, etc.; KCS in shih tzu's, Lhasas, etc. Using the breed search mode of your computer you should be able to identify breeds and ages of your client's pets. Develop an educational letter about a specific problem, e.g., thyroid disease. List its breed predilection and the clinical signs seen and make them an offer they can't refuse. For example a free thyroid check with a full profile; one month's free Soloxine with low thyroid; etc. Then, tell them about the packages that you have for dogs with hypothyroidism (see above).

Train to Trust

For each program, package, ratio, etc., the doctors and paraprofessionals all have to be on the same page of the program. Staff meetings are imperative to implement and then troubleshoot these programs. I love role playing between the doctor and client using the staff members as clients and paraprofessionals.

Have your paraprofessionals contribute their input to the client education/marketing pieces. Remember you are selling these packages to clients who may not be well versed on preventative healthcare themselves.

These programs are presented to clients in multiple fashions:

Mailers to selected pets and clients—use your computer to search and sort or create links to reminders.

Over the phone when a client calls—"Mrs. Smith, have you heard about our new skin care programs for your itchy dog designed to be more thorough in addressing your pet's condition and more affordable for you? Can I fax you a copy prior to your visit?"

In the exam room after the OPN checks in the client, an appropriate brochure or handout can be left for the client to peruse.

It is imperative that the paraprofessional completely understand the scope of the programs. They must support them 100 percent. They must understand the medicine behind the marketing. They must believe that these programs will present a benefit to the pet, the client, and most importantly to the practice and thus to themselves.

Consider rewarding either the entire staff or individual staff members for packages that are purchased. Set monthly goals. Compare similar months from year to year for trends. Have the staff review the handouts regularly for needed changes. Let them know that the packages are theirs too.

The Computer

How does your computer fit into the package? You must learn how to use your computer to create simple single code bundle entries. By entering one code number, you create an entire list of procedures and reminders and an attached package price (see Appendix 2).

Secondly, you must use your computer to track your monthly procedure counts and ratios. How many packages were purchased? How many ear smears did you do? What is your kitten exam to FeLV test ratio?

Based on historical information, how many of each package or procedure should you be performing each day, week, or month? How can you increase this number?

Also, take advantage of your database. Search and sort. How many unspayed female dogs or cats do you have? What about a spay/neuter reminder? When was the last dental procedure done on your eight-year-old dogs or cats? Remember the breed predilection discussion? This is where the computer starts to earn you some bucks.

Other Points to Ponder

Do you remember to run urinalysis with your profiles? Do you know that the urine specific gravity might be an earlier indication of renal damage than either the BUN or creatinine? Include this with *all* lab work as part of your screens. Most labs will create a custom profile to your specifications, including a urinalysis and/or T4 with your most commonly run profile. Do you think that you can truly regulate a diabetic with a single blood glucose? How many times can you collect blood from a diabetic cat before he collects blood from you? Purchase a human glucosometer. You can do one-drop blood glucose levels every one to two hours throughout the day and start to get a true measure of the changes before you adjust your insulin levels or start using glycosolated hemoglobin on fractious cats and neurotic dogs. What percentage of your anesthetic procedures receives lab work? If it's not 100 percent, what do you need to do increase compliance? Remember the two yes answers from Chapter Two. What about IV catheters?

By creating programs and procedures that are standards for your practice you will:

✓ allow the team to buy in,
✓ allow the clients to see the quality you provide,
✓ define the patient needs,
✓ provide more consistent care, and
✓ increase profitability.

Inpatient Procedures 4

When to Admit for Day Care

In Chapter Three we discussed the concept of quality time and the client's desire to spend less than 20 minutes in the exam room. So how do we accomplish extended workups that include radiographs, EKGs, ultrasounds, and other diagnostics? It's called the day admit. Within your 10 minutes of time with the pet a decision is made that a workup will be required. At that point you state the need to the client and put a box in the medical records. You establish a callback or pickup time with the client and turn the patient over to the inpatient team as discussed below. Anything requiring more than the allotted time in the appointment book goes to the back. A quick blood draw for CBC and chemistry panel or urinalysis can be done while the client is being invoiced. Anything more extensive requires a day admit.

Our practice draws people from several hours away. We offer "yes" alternatives: Go get some lunch; board the pet overnight; go shopping in Reno; or wait up front and watch the fish tank. A practice in Canada made a deal with the diner next door to give the client a coupon good for a piece of pie. Another idea is to issue your clients a pager. They can go shopping, out to lunch, or to the car wash. When Ralph is ready, you page them. They don't need to sit by a phone all day. When they pick Ralph up, they return the pager. Be creative and responsive to your client's needs without stressing your staff by making unrealistic promises.

The White Board—Backend Salvation

So far we've concentrated on the exam room and the front door. Now to the heart of the practice. No, not the computer, the treatment room. Two very important topics are teamwork and the white board. Let's discuss the simple one first. Figure 4.1 is the treatment room white board when one board is divided for medical procedures and treatments of hospitalized patients. In the good old days it was a chalkboard; we still have a big one. Nowadays most folks have two or three erasable marker boards in their treatment room. Figure 4.2 is a surgery/anesthetic board. You can use one for surgery, one for all other procedures, and one for treatments. You can combine one or more by splitting the board in half.

Practices with big boarding business keep a separate one for heartworm and boarding medications, kennel assignments, baths, and special packages. See Chapter Five for kennel use. Necessary columns include date/Dr/patient/Rx or procedure for those two boards. Treatment board needs date/Dr/. You guessed it, boxes for s.i.d., b.i.d., t.i.d. that get initialed when done. At the end of the day, the closing tech or assistant transfers the white board to the medical record and starts tomorrow's boards with patients still in the hospital. Some practices then do daily charge outs while completing the medical record. This is also sometimes done during the noontime lull. A circle sheet is done at the same time.

FIGURE 4.1

WHITE BOARD FOR PROCEDURES AND TREATMENTS

Date	Pet	Owner	Procedure	Doctor	Date	Pet	Owner	Treatment
10/11/98	Murphy	Cole	x-ray abdm	Ross	10/11/98	Max	Crider	T4 [ ] [ ]
10/11/98	Missy	Hex	CBC/Chem	Haig	10/11/98	Moses	Rebar	Ceph250 [ ] [ ] [ ]

FIGURE 4.2

WHITE BOARD FOR SURGERY/ANESTHESIA

Date	Pet	Owner	Surgery	Preop	IV TKO	Full IV
11/12/98	Riya	Hanson	OFA	no	no	no
	Max	Hendrikson	OHE	1	yes	
	Hope	McCauley	Fx Pelvis	4		yes

Teamwork

Now comes the fun part—teamwork. In a busy practice, using our system, traffic flow is a beauty to behold. I came from a doctor-intensive practice, an "I could do it all and nobody could do it better" background. I was very proud of my ability to do everything without assistants. Boy was I stupid! Let's run one of our day admit patients through the system. The doctor–outpatient team has boxed the needs, i.e., the diagnostic plan, in the medical records. The doctor or outpatient nurse has brought the patient to the treatment room. Here's the first set of alternatives in a hospital with a team. Everybody in back is busy. The OPN puts the patient into a kennel, labels the patient and kennel, writes the procedure on the appropriate white board, and puts the record in the To Do slot. In the second alternative the intake tech or assistant is not busy, but the exam rooms are humming. They take the pet and do as above. The doctor can also perform this function if everyone else is occupied.

Now I need to digress a moment to discuss staffing. This paragraph will save you a ton of money. Almost every practice we go into for the first time is top heavy. Doctors are doing tech work, techs are doing assistant work, and assistants are doing kennel work. What? Four levels of employees in the back room of a veterinary hospital? Kennel help cleans cages morning and evening. They can also mop floors, empty trash, and restock shelves. In a small practice they can move forward to be trained as an assistant during midday. Assistants hold animals, take x-rays, give subcutaneous fluids and injections, hang fluids, prep surgeries, clean and polish teeth, and assist technicians. Technicians draw blood, give anesthetics, give IV injections and place catheters, do dental extractions, and run the back end. So what do doctors do? Diagnose, prescribe, do surgery, and talk to clients. Nirvana!

Here comes the ton of savings. If you are a typical practice, you can increase your productivity tremendously by hiring from the bottom up. Hire a minimum wage kennel caretaker, i.e., a high school student. That's right, with today's flex scheduling, students are available mornings and evenings. The next step is to hire and train an assistant. To start with they're taught restraint. Then they are trained in other procedures during staff training meetings and on the job. There is another beauty to this system that may not be apparent. It's self-perpetuating. We have assistants and receptionists who have been with us since high school. I have a receptionist in veterinary school and two assistants in prevet!

I will use a large practice to illustrate alternative number one for simplicity. In a smaller practice these teams may, in fact, all be one team. Team one is the surgery team. We have a surgery tech with two assistants. The surgery tech or surgery doctor (Let go and let the team do its job!) prioritizes the cases for the day. The tech anesthetizes patients, places IVs, and does medical records for routine cases. The tech may also charge out routine cases. Assistant one preps animals and moves them into surgery. Assistant two recovers the surgical patient. What does the doctor do? Change gloves until surgery is done. The team also calls each client as soon as the patient is either finished or recovered and schedules a pickup time.

Team two has two variations. We'll call it the intake tech and inpatient team. The real variation is whether or not it includes a doctor. If a single doctor follows cases all the way through, then we have an intake tech with an assistant. If the doctor writes up a treatment and/or diagnostic plan and turns it over to the inpatient doctor, we have a tech with two assistants. Just to confuse you further, the a.m. outpatient doctor can rotate to the p.m. inpatient doctor to follow cases. The key difference here is walk-ins. If there is an inpatient doctor, this is who sees walk-ins. If not, there are gray areas in the appointment book, which are appointments not booked until that day. The rest of the team's duties are as follows. The assistants hold dogs, take x-rays, and perform other duties as listed above. The tech draws blood, places catheters, gives IV injections, calculates flow rates for fluids, and runs the rest of the treatment room not concerning surgery. The tech is the boss when you have multiple doctors all wanting their patient cared for first. The white board is used to prioritize procedures and inform everyone about what's going on already. If a doctor walks back with a patient for a quick x-ray while the owner waits, and there are six already waiting for x-rays, guess what? Day admit! Don't harass the intake tech unless the pet is dying!

The final inpatient team is the dental team. That's right, if you're not doing enough dentistries to require a separate team, read about dental programs below. This team requires a tech and an assistant. The dental tech anesthetizes patients, places IVs, checks the assistant's work, and does extractions. The tech can also assist the intake and/or surgery tech if necessary. The assistant cleans, polishes, and recovers the dental patient.

The dental tech replaces the surgery tech for lunch. The dental tech and surgery tech can obviously be the same person. A single tech can also do all three jobs. Modify the above examples to fit your practice. Dentistry in the a.m. can be followed by surgery at noon. Use the wet table for doing dentistry while the doctor is in surgery. The variables are endless. The real key to maximum production is simple. Techs don't do assistant work; doctors don't do tech work. But remember, it's a team. I clean kennels and mop floors on occasion. I draw blood or urine once a week. I even put in an IV catheter now and then. Get the picture? It's a wonderful way to practice. We have adapted Tom Cat's methods to our practice. We are located in rural Nevada. We don't have fleas or heartworms. All my partners produce the numbers Tom preaches, and I feel semiretired compared to the old way. Peter practices in Orange County, California. He gets the same results in a radically different practice environment. Just imagine how many more clients you could see and what a better job you could do by eliminating all that tech work you're personally doing.

Dental Programs

Now that we have our teams in place, what programs can we do with all this extra time and help? The most obvious starting place is dental. It's 90 percent staff work, it's highly profitable, and most of our patients need it. Start by grading teeth. Use the CET or similar brochure to standardize all the OPNs, doctors, and techs. Have your OPNs include grading teeth as part of their wellness exam outlined in Chapter Two. Then establish different prices for each grade. Grade I are those dentals most of us aren't doing. Sometimes they're called juvenile prophys. Anesthetic, cleaning and polishing, at the time of publication, should be around $75. This will vary by location and current pricing structure. Remember, this is all assistant work and really quick turnaround. Conflict arises with your anesthetic charges. This is probably what you charge for Isoflurane now. Remember, this is a really quick procedure. It probably takes less than 20 minutes. If you get into the habit of doing these, it's better for the pet and the net! Grade II dentals should probably cost about what you're charging now. Plus or minus $100 would be in the ballpark. If you're in a price-sensitive, competitive area, stay under $100.

To make the numbers work, many practices have Prophy I, II, III, and IV and Dental Anesthetic I, II, III, and IV. Grades 3 and 4 are much higher and to some degree are governed by how you charge for extractions. You could include finger pulls, charge by tooth, or charge by time. I recommend that you quote for antibiotics and pain medication separately. Some practices include this all in one fee. Don't forget all those protocols from Chapter Three. You should have one for each grade including preanesthetic blood work, IV TKO, and pain medication. The higher grades would add extractions, antibiotics, and higher levels of diagnostics if the patient is geriatric. See Appendix 1 for sample dental programs by grade.

A really fun addition to the overall dental plan is called dental contesting. The specifics are tailored to the practice, but here are the general principles. First, start with general training programs to cover the basics of grading, cleaning, polishing, and simple extractions for the assistants and technicians. Then send your staff to one of the many continuing education opportunities for dental education. Ideally send them to a program with a wet lab. Now comes the fun (scary) part. Let them pick out your next dental unit. This is especially important if you are not yet polishing teeth or using a high-speed hand piece for splitting teeth. Now look at your numbers and set a goal for the quarter. If you double the number of dentals, or some other realistic increase, for a quarter, then you can be assured of the income necessary to pay for the new unit. It's a win-win situation. The staff gets educated and gets a new "toy"; you get new equipment for the clinic. And it's all funded by increased production!

Now let's continue to grow your dental practice. Free outpatient exams for dental grading are done by OPNs, not doctors. Follow-up appointments for home care, brushing, T/D sales, CET Chews, and other dental products are all done by your dental hygiene specialist. Time to send you to continuing education with a wet lab, or better still send an associate. Let's start treating those periodontal lesions, maybe even a root canal or two. Really excited? What about orthodontics, caps, and crowns? There are practices out there with veterinarians doing only dentistry! There are no limits to the income potential and most of it is still staff time! This is really an opportunity to increase the net with minimal doctor time.

Geriatric Programs

Do you have a senior friends program? At what age do you start it? How about planting the seed with that first heartworm test or anesthetic procedure. "Ms. Duzan, Dr. Cole recommends a baseline blood panel to establish normal values for Talak. These tests will increase with age as we begin to screen for geriatric problems. For now he recommends starting with XYZ. Would you like me to include that with his heartworm test since we're drawing blood anyway?" Similar dialogue is used for the first anesthetic procedure and screening for birth defects, especially of the liver and kidneys. Most labs have profiles already set up for different age groups, or you can define your own. See if it's more economical and/or quicker to run in-house.

Now build from there based on your beliefs. What's appropriate for a dog or cat less than two years old? QBC or CBC or just a PCV? Clotting time, ACT? Urine specific gravity with a dipstick or a full UA? BUN, Creatinine, ALT, or SAP? Now what about from two to six or eight? Top end of all the above? Full chemistry panel? What about over eight? All the above plus chest and abdominal x-rays? ECG? Ultrasound? Multiple levels of geriatric exams can cover from ages six to 20 depending on the individual's health and age. Make sure your staff knows your values, and many of these exams will be presold at the front desk or in the exam room. You define your comfort zone and then train the staff. Remember that preventative medicine is recognized and demanded by today's consumer. See Appendix 1 and Chapter 1 for more information on developing your programs.

Hospitalization

Next let's define your hospitalization program. Hospitalization requires huge amounts of staff time. There are basically two schools of thought on how to adequately charge for that time. The first is to charge for everything you do individually. This certainly is sound thinking, but in the rush of charge out, items are often missed. One way to avoid this is to use and review the protocols in Chapter Two. The second school of thought is to establish four levels of care. Define what's included, and charge accordingly. At the simplest level, frequency of treatment can be used. s.i.d, b.i.d., t.i.d., and q.i.d. each require a different degree of staff time. Do you include the pill or charge for medication in addition? Another way to look at levels of care is the degree of difficulty or expertise required to administer the treatment. Level one is oral. Level two is IM and SQ injections and fluid. Level 3 is IV injections and fluids. Level 4 includes intensive care monitoring. Again the price will depend on what medications are included and which ones are charged out separately.

Now that you have your staff trained, your protocols and hospitalization charges in place, and your programs defined, how do you monitor your progress? A diagnostic to pharmacy ratio is a simple way to find out if you are practicing good quality diagnostics or just pushing pills. Although it will vary with each hospital, the trend and the difference between doctors is valid within that hospital. Don't make it hard. Take your x-ray, ultrasound, and lab categories from your veterinary computer and divide it by the total dispensed medication. This will give you a starting point for your practice. The closer to 1:1 the number is, the better your diagnostic procedures are.

Next measure your state-of-the-art procedures. Ultrasounds, tonopen measurements, blood pressure, endoscopy, and otoscopy are just a few. If you start any new procedure from those to acupuncture, track it and make sure you didn't just buy a new toy and get bored with it. Another area that's critical to monitor is your lab expense. How much should you do in-house versus at an outside lab? There are two areas to consider: service and price. With the massive consolidation of laboratories, many of us don't really have a choice any more for basic support. In some cases support has improved and in others it's worse. What's your turnaround time? Most of us have to do same-day pre-ops in-house. What about critical patient monitoring? At what point does it pay to invest in the people and equipment necessary to run a full in-house lab? Often that answer is determined more by service than by cost. During the conversion to whatever point you decide, monitor both in-house lab, send-out lab, and total lab. Monitor costs, gross sales, and procedures to make sure that the level of care doesn't fall or costs exceed charges.

Your computer can easily track any or all of the above examples. Look at our dozen dots and procedure charting in Appendix G of Volume 2. Add or subtract from these depending on your current emphasis. Look at procedure counts and total dollars per category or line item. If you are doing program-based budgeting, then you'll know if a particular area is paying for itself. Once you have decided what to monitor this quarter or year, set goals for improvement. Once your goals are set, involve the appropriate staff member(s) in tracking the progress. This sends the message that these goals are important to you and that their efforts are being monitored and appreciated. Ideally we have tied a staff reward to either the individual program or overall hospital performance. Now let's talk about the rest of our chores.

Busywork by Position—A New Scheduling Concept

We all have those jobs that are essential to running a practice, but not immediate emergencies. They often never get done until December of every year or just before closing or maybe once a week.

Our first checklist is for those slow times when the receptionist really can't leave the front desk, but shouldn't just gossip or read *People* magazine:

Receptionist Chores to Do When It's Slow

- ❏ Go through magazines in exam rooms/waiting room and throw away any dog-eared or very old ones.
- ❏ Straighten bulletin board; throw away anything over 2 months old; date all existing postings.
- ❏ Straighten picture board, take down any puppy or kitten pictures more than 3 months old and put them in client chart to be given to client.
- ❏ Go through drawers and cupboards—clean, straighten, check for low stock to put on want list.
- ❏ Put together kitten and puppy kits.
- ❏ Go through client handouts; throw away any that are faded or wrinkled. Make additional copies if needed.
- ❏ Go through client brochures/pamphlets in drawer—straighten; put on want list if low.
- ❏ Restock, clean, and straighten both pharmacies.
- ❏ Clean, restock canned dog and cat foods.
- ❏ Clean, restock treats display.
- ❏ Restock leashes and collars.
- ❏ Use Equalizer cleaner on any stained or soiled chairs.

❑ Move everything off counters and dust/clean behind and under things.

❑ Go through cremations and call any clients that have been over 2 months since last call.

❑ Clean wall where back of chairs touch in waiting room.

❑ Check weekly and daily maintenance lists.

❑ Clean baseboards around floor area.

❑ Dust/clean mini blinds.

❑ Wash walls in waiting room, front hallway, and exam rooms.

Like everything else, these are only ideas to stimulate you to think about what needs to be done in your practice. After you have created the list and the staff members are yakking, the supervisor merely reminds them that the list needs to be done before anybody leaves for the day. The same thing occurs when it's slow and someone wants to go home. Ask, "Is the list done yet?"

Who has the final responsibility to pull files, send sympathy cards, and put away today's files? What do I mean by final responsibility? That person doesn't get to go home until it's done. Our practice manager and her technician team recently initiated a maintenance checklist. Here's their version of what needs to be done daily, weekly, and monthly:

DAILY MAINTENANCE CHECKLIST

Surgery Room—ST/SA (Surgery tech/Surgery assistant)
- ❏ Spot clean walls (esp. blood stains)
- ❏ Clean surgical tables (esp. bases)
- ❏ Clean all surfaces
- ❏ Clean anesthesia machine (incl. valves)
- ❏ Chg. Baralyme grans. (as needed)—post date
- ❏ Close doors to surgery when done

Radiology Room—IT (Intake tech)
- ❏ Clean and straighten aprons & gloves
- ❏ Wipe down x-ray table (esp. sides)
- ❏ Check levels of developing fluids
- ❏ Spot clean walls

Dental Room—DT/TA (Dental tech/treatment assistant)
- ❏ Clean behind tub (in corner)
- ❏ Clean & wipe down dental machine
- ❏ Scrub & wash tub (esp. sides/bases)
- ❏ Chg. Baralyme grans. (as needed)—post date
- ❏ Spot clean walls

Laboratory—IT
- ❏ Wipe down counters (all surfaces)
- ❏ Wipe down all machines
- ❏ Scrub sink
- ❏ Spot clean walls

Exam Rooms #1, 2, 3, 4, 5, 6—OPN (Dr.'s asst.)

Clean chairs/tables	❏	❏	❏	❏	❏	❏
Clean/organize shelves	❏	❏	❏	❏	❏	❏
Remove hair	❏	❏	❏	❏	❏	❏
Scrub sinks	❏	❏	❏	❏	❏	❏
Clean tables (top & base)	❏	❏	❏	❏	❏	❏
Wipe down counters	❏	❏	❏	❏	❏	❏
Refill all solutions	❏	❏	❏	❏	❏	❏
Restock paper towels	❏	❏	❏	❏	❏	❏
Chg. ear cone soln.	❏	❏	❏	❏	❏	❏
Check cold trays (chg. PRN)	❏	❏	❏	❏	❏	❏
Spot clean walls	❏	❏	❏	❏	❏	❏
Restock syringes	❏	❏	❏	❏	❏	❏
Wipe down pharmacy counters	❏	❏				
Scrub sink in pharmacy #1	❏					

Breakroom—On Call
- ❏ Wash dishes
- ❏ Wipe down counter tops
- ❏ Clean table/chairs
- ❏ Spot clean walls

Treatment Room—DT/TA
- ❏ Clean all tables (esp. sides/bases)
- ❏ Refill fluids

WEEKLY MAINTENANCE CHECKLIST

Surgery Room
- ❏ Clean door tops, doors, & counters
- ❏ Dust cobwebs
- ❏ Restock suture/organize cupboards
- ❏ Clean window, sill, & blinds
- ❏ Disinfect hoses & bags
- ❏ Clean surgical lamps

Radiology Room
- ❏ Wipe down film bin/control panel
- ❏ Clean door tops & door
- ❏ Wipe down processor (inside/out)
- ❏ Dust cobwebs
- ❏ Clean & organize shelves
- ❏ Clean view box
- ❏ Clean processor shelf
- ❏ Clean tray under x-ray table
- ❏ Wash muzzles

Laboratory
- ❏ Clean centrifuges (under/behind etc.)
- ❏ Dust cobwebs
- ❏ Clean/organize shelves & cabinets
- ❏ Check lab supplies
- ❏ Clean bottles & containers
- ❏ Restock shelves & drawers

Breakroom
- ❏ Clean door & windowsill
- ❏ Dust cobwebs
- ❏ Clean inside & outside of refrigerator

Dental Room
- ❏ Clean/organize drawers & cabinet
- ❏ Wipe down push cart shelves
- ❏ Clean supplies on turntable etc.
- ❏ Change cold tray fluid
- ❏ Wipe off gas anesthesia machine
- ❏ Autoclave instruments in cold tray
- ❏ Change cold tray solution

continued

WEEKLY MAINTENANCE CHECKLIST *continued*

Treatment Room
- ☐ Clean chalkboard
- ☐ Clean autoclave (w/solution)
- ☐ Organize & stock drawers/cabinets/shelves
- ☐ Dust cobwebs
- ☐ Clean out cabinets under sink
- ☐ Clean prep table lights
- ☐ Change cold tray solution w/disinfectant
- ☐ Clean doors & tops
- ☐ Autoclave instruments in cold tray
- ☐ Fill Vaseline containers
- ☐ Clean refrigerator (in & out)

Pharmacy 1 & 2

Clean/restock shelves/drawers/cabinets	☐	☐
Dust pictures & remove cobwebs	☐	☐
Spot clean all walls	☐	☐
Clean doors & tops	☐	☐
Clean refrigerator (in & out)	☐	☐
Restock pill vials	☐	☐
Wipe down computer & printer	☐	☐

Examination Room #1, 2, 3, 4, 5, 6

Change thermometer container w/Benz-all	☐	☐	☐	☐	☐	☐
Dust pictures & remove cobwebs	☐	☐	☐	☐	☐	☐
Change cold tray solution	☐	☐	☐	☐	☐	☐
Fill Vaseline containers	☐	☐	☐	☐	☐	☐
Clean doors & frames	☐	☐	☐	☐	☐	☐

MONTHLY MAINTENANCE CHECKLIST

Surgery Room
- ❏ Clean & oil cabinet fronts
- ❏ Test emergency light
- ❏ Vacuum air vents
- ❏ Clean baseboards
- ❏ Clean & check light fixtures

Laboratory
- ❏ Clean microscope
- ❏ Clean & check light fixtures
- ❏ Clean & oil cabinet fronts
- ❏ Clean baseboards
- ❏ Vacuum air vent
- ❏ Calibrate vet test machine
- ❏ Check expiration dates on supplies

Radiology Room
- ❏ Clean & check light fixtures
- ❏ Clean baseboards
- ❏ Vacuum air vents

Dental Room
- ❏ Clean & check light fixtures
- ❏ Clean baseboards
- ❏ Vacuum air vent

Examination Rooms #1, 2, 3, 4, 5, 6

Vacuum air vents	❏	❏	❏	❏	❏	❏
Clean baseboards	❏	❏	❏	❏	❏	❏
Clean & check light fixtures	❏	❏	❏	❏	❏	❏

Treatment Room
- ❏ Clean & check light fixtures
- ❏ Defrost freezer
- ❏ Clean & oil cabinets
- ❏ Clean glass cabinets (inside & out)
- ❏ Clean prep table lights
- ❏ Vacuum air vents
- ❏ Resterilize outdated packs & instruments
- ❏ Clean baseboards

continued

MONTHLY MAINTENANCE CHECKLIST *continued*

Breakroom
- ❑ Clean baseboards
- ❑ Clean & check light fixtures
- ❑ Vacuum air vents

Pharmacy 1 & 2

Clean & oil cabinets	❑	❑
Defrost freezer	❑	❑
Clean & check light fixtures	❑	❑
Clean baseboards	❑	❑
Vacuum air vents	❑	❑

Kennel Area
- ❑ Clean & check light fixtures
- ❑ Vacuum air vents
- ❑ Clean exhaust fans
- ❑ Clean baseboards
- ❑ Check & repair gates & hardware

If everything wasn't done during the week, the Saturday crew does not get to go home until it's done. Tuesday afternoon before Christmas the place was a cleaning zoo! Heather assigns those jobs by title and schedule position. In other words it isn't always Carrie's job. It's the opening or closing receptionist's responsibility. Or it's the a.m. or p.m. assistant's job. It's the surgery tech or the intake tech. Everything from drug logs to changing soda lime canisters has someone or some position assigned to do it. In our practice the opening lists and closing lists are broken down to the reception area, the treatment room, and the kennel caretakers. Our daily lists cover things that must be done that day to keep the hospital clean, running well, and the animals cared for. The weekly maintenance lists and monthly maintenance lists help us remember things like changing air filters, oiling cabinet fronts, and defrosting freezers. Our technicians even developed a maintenance log so that they could communicate with each other on the status of various equipment repairs. See Figure 4.3.

The opening receptionist procedures include the usual: make sure the waiting area is clean and ready for clients; count the beginning money and put it in the money drawer; boot up the computers; turn on the copy machine; distribute the lab work with charts that came during the night; and take the phones off call forwarding. The ultimate responsibility for ensuring that the waiting room and exam rooms are clean and ready for clients lies with the opening receptionist. In our area we get snow and ice during the winter, so the responsibility of making sure the "caution wet floor" signs are out and the walkway is shoveled is the opening receptionist's as well. The receptionist doesn't have to shovel the walk or put the signs out if there is a kennel assistant to delegate to, but does have to make sure it is done. Our receptionist responsibilities are assigned according to shifts. During the day the receptionist answering the phone is responsible for pulling all the next day's charts as well as for reviewing then filing today's charts. The receptionist who greets clients is responsible for calling all the next day's appointments to confirm. The receptionist who loads exam rooms and fills medications is responsible for delivering messages, keeping the pharmacy in order and ensuring that the precounted medicine drawers are filled, posting updated appointment schedules, and distributing lab work. The receptionist who processes invoices and checks people out is responsible for all the closing procedures. All of them work on our welcome and sympathy cards during the slow times.

MAINTENANCE AND REPAIR LOG

Date	Problem	Reported by	Who was called	Phone #	Estimated date fixed

FIGURE 4.3

The closer cannot leave, however, until these jobs are done. There is a great deal of peer pressure to get your jobs done so the closer doesn't have to stay until midnight doing everything.

The closing receptionist prints the next day's recall list and pulls charts to be distributed to the appropriate doctor, technician, or receptionist for the phone call. This person is also responsible for printing the end-of-the-day money sheets, counting and balancing the money, and doing the computer backup. The closing receptionist is ultimately responsible for making sure all files are filed, new client labels typed, sympathy and welcome cards done, recalls done, and the reception area clean and ready for the next day.

Our opening animal assistant is responsible for morning TPR; notation of urine, stool and appetite; and treatments. This person must review all medical files and check all patients in the hospital. This is done with the help of our morning kennel assistant. By 7 a.m. when the next shift arrives this should all be done, files completed, and a patient status list taken to the receptionists. The opening assistant is also responsible for turning on the x-ray processor and lab equipment. Our midday treatments are ultimately the responsibility of the intake technician, although the assistant to the doctor handling the case often does them. Cleaning and restocking the exam rooms as well as their cold trays falls to each doctor's assistant. The evening treatments and charting are the responsibility of the closing assistant or technician, although the doctor's assistant often does these as well. Our team in the treatment room works very well together to make sure all tasks are completed and no one gets dumped on. The closing assistant/technician is responsible for seeing that all animals are treated, are comfortable, and their charts are updated. This person is also responsible for turning off the equipment, making sure all packs and instruments are autoclaved for the next day, making sure laundry is done, etc. He/she also signs off the kennel assistant's checklist for the day.

Here's the checklist to get you started:

CLOSING CHECKLIST FOR TREATMENT

1. All treatments given and charted ❑
2. Animals have food, water, blanket, and litter box (if cat) ❑
3. Check all medical records ❑
4. Horses locked up ❑
5. Restock and clean ❑
6. 6 packs autoclaved ❑
   2 stockinettes of each size (sm, med, lg) autoclaved ❑
   6 gauze packs autoclaved ❑
   Ellman unit instruments gas sterilized ❑
   4 towel packs autoclaved ❑
   2 large green drapes autoclaved ❑
   4 gowns autoclaved ❑
   Any specialty instruments autoclaved ❑
   6¼" and 6½" Penrose drains autoclaved ❑
   12 pup rugs washed, dried, folded, and put away ❑
7. All x-rays put away ❑
   Stickers put on x-ray folders of hospitalized animals ❑
   No x-rays loose ❑
8. IDEXX analyzer off and covered ❑
9. Microscope off and covered ❑
10. Put away and lock up controlled drugs ❑
11. Counters clean and area neat ❑
12. Laundry done and machines turned off ❑
13. Sign kennel caretaker's checklist ❑
14. Fecals done, recorded in chart, and owner notified ❑
15. Equipment, boxes, etc. left outside put away ❑
16. Refrigerated items unpacked and put away ❑
17. Anesthetic machines unplugged, etc. ❑
18. Turn off main oxygen outside ❑
19. Check all cold trays ❑
20. Restock fluids and drip sets ❑
21. Coffeepot and toaster unplugged ❑
22. Turn off lights except hallways ❑
23. Write pager # and home # on treatment board ❑
24. Double-check that all doors and windows/blinds are closed ❑
25. Turn off air conditioner/make sure heater is set ❑
26. Autoclave is turned off ❑
27. Front cages closed and have a clip on them ❑
28. FeLV Saliva test refrigerated ❑
29. Turn on alarm system if you are the last one out ❑
30. Turn compressor off, bleed line, & leave open ❑
31. Stock fluids in incubator ❑
32. Oil & clean (w/toothbrush) all clipper blades on clippers ❑
33. Change ear cone solution w/Benz-all ❑

Signature:_____ Date:_____

Note the places for dates and signatures. No finger-pointing or say-ing, "It ain't my job." If a task isn't performed properly on the week-end, the manager knows whose responsibility it was. Even if dele-gated, it's one person's responsibility to ensure that the task was performed.

Our daily tasks in the treatment area are broken down by position. Our surgery doctor for the day has a team of the surgery technician, surgery assistant, dental technician and dental assistant. The surgery tech and assistant work together to pre-op, anesthetize, and prep all surgeries. (The surgery doctor scrubs in and goes from surgery to surgery.) The dental technician and dental assistant work together to pre-op, anesthetize, and complete all dental procedures. The intake technician is available to all the doctors besides the surgery doctor for the day. The doctors have their own unlicensed animal assistant assigned to them for the day. This person works as an outpatient nurse in the exam rooms and completing procedures with the intake technician in the back. The intake technician works with the doctor's assistants to prioritize procedures on the treatment board and to make sure they are done. Together they do all the blood draws, catheter placement and fluid therapy, radiographs, lab work, and anything that does not require a doctor. All busywork is done ac-cording to the day's position assignment. When the surgery crew is done, they clean up that area; maintain the anesthetic machines; and clean and autoclave the packs, gowns, and instruments. When the dental crew is done, they clean and maintain the dental room, the dentistry machine, and the anesthetic machine. The intake technician keeps an eye on the treatment room for cleanliness all day. The doc-tor's assistants are responsible for their exam rooms and any mess they make in treatment.

OSHA compliance is also a group effort. We hold an annual staff training meeting. The practice manager divides the staff into teams then lets them choose safety topics out of a hat. Each team then pre-pares a presentation for the rest of the staff on that safety topic, which they present at our annual meeting. The meeting is videotaped and shown to anyone who could not be there and to all new hires throughout the year. Ongoing OSHA topics are presented in the newsletter employees receive with their paychecks. Any refresher ar-eas that are needed can be covered in our monthly staff meetings. The MSDS maintenance is the responsibility of our purchasing manager.

The Control Drug Log is maintained monthly by one of our technicians and reviewed by the practice manager. Repairs and major equipment maintenance are the ultimate responsibility of another technician. Initial and ongoing training falls to yet another technician. A different technician assists the practice manager in interviewing and screening new applicants. The technicians rotate responsibilities once every six months or so.

The kennel caretakers also have an opening and closing list of tasks. On the next page is an example of the closing list that the closing assistant mentioned above has to sign off:

KENNEL CARETAKER DAILY CHECKLIST

Afternoon

1. Check all animals at the beginning of your shift ❏
   (front and back kennel)
2. Check reception area at the beginning of your shift and hourly ❏
3. Clean all cages and runs (make sure runs are draining) ❏
4. Let all dogs out in the exercise run (check gate first) ❏
5. Clean up exercise run between each dog and when done ❏
6. Place clean, dry blankets in all cages ❏
7. Place litter boxes in all cat's cages (yesterday's news if declaw) ❏
8. Water and feed animals ❏
9. Fill out all boxes on cage cards w/pertinent information (both) ❏
10. Check isolation room daily ❏
11. Wash food and water dishes and put away. Clean counter ❏
12. Empty all garbage (make sure can is empty) when you leave ❏
13. Sweep and mop kennel (change mop water) room floors ❏
14. Make sure kennel tub is clean and free of hair ❏
15. Scrub cage doors and grates ❏
16. Clean surgery room ❏
17. Put away deliveries ❏
18. Empty poop bucket and replace liner ❏
19. Scrub treatment tubs and counters/scrub dental tub ❏
20. Restock treatment area and exam rooms ❏
21. Scrub exam room counters ❏
22. Make at least 12 cat boxes before leaving ❏
23. Clean surgical packs and put up to be autoclaved ❏
24. Plug in otoscopes at end of night ❏
25. Keep laundry running (done before you leave) ❏
26. Clean kitchen/break room ❏
27. Restock front bathroom ❏
28. Check all animals immediately before leaving ❏
29. Check kennel area immediately before leaving ❏
30. Make sure kennel door is locked and shut tightly ❏

On Saturdays

1. **Do first**—clean stalls/corrals, make sure horses have water ❏
   (clean stalls on Sunday too)
2. Scrub laundry baskets ❏
3. Clean drains and prep sinks ❏
4. Clean hair out of vacuum canister ❏
5. Flush x-ray drain. Make sure water is turned back on ❏
6. Vacuum and mop entire hospital before leaving ❏
7. Check lawn, front entry, and parking lot for litter and stool ❏
8. Clean freezer ❏

Date:

Kennel Caretaker:_____Assistant/Tech:_____

Our opening caretaker is responsible for cleaning, exercising, and feeding all animals as well as helping the morning treatment assistant with TPR and treatments. This caretaker is responsible for keeping an eye on all the animals all morning. She puts clean, warm blankets in cages in preparation for post-op patients. She is responsible for making sure no animal sits in a mess, but that they get cleaned immediately. She also keeps up on cleaning the surgical packs and getting them autoclaved so they don't run out during the busy surgical schedule. She is the one the receptionists call for a wet clean-up, for assistance bringing a patient in, or to take food to someone's car. She keeps the laundry running and helps keep the treatment area clean as well. Her ultimate responsibility lies with the animals and keeping them clean and comfortable. The closing kennel caretaker also cleans, exercises, and feeds. This caretaker must also restock the treatment area, empty all garbage, have the laundry done before leaving, put together disposable cat litter boxes, mop the surgery room, and perform all the end-of-the-day kennel procedures. Both caretakers assist with completing the daily, weekly, and monthly checklists for hospital maintenance.

Look around your practice and every time you find a necessary, boring, repetitive job not getting done, assign it on a regularly scheduled basis. Assign it by job description and schedule position. Better yet, sit down with your team and have them make lists of their pet peeves. Have them decide what needs to be done. While all of you are brainstorming you can throw in your ideas to make sure they end up on the list as well. But the ultimate result will be their ideas, not yours. Ask them who has the ultimate responsibility. Once they have made the list and the rules, they will make it work. After all, you did not dictate it to them, so they will be responsible for it. Our technicians police our maintenance lists regularly. None of them has any more authority than any other one, so they all encourage and scold one another until it gets done. Now when it is slow and someone wants to go home early, their peers say, "Is everything done on the monthly checklist?" They chat with each other while cleaning and checking off items on their list rather than standing around. Only once has the practice manager had to post the unfinished list in the treatment room with the question "Why weren't these checked off?" The staff has complimented each other on what a great job they have done keeping up on the lists. They comment on how the hospital is so much cleaner than it used to be. They take pride in what they have accomplished on their own. The entire hospital functions on teamwork and cooperation. The checklists and job assignments ensure that all the maintenance and boring chores don't fall to one person, but still get accomplished with minimal nagging.

Marketing 5

For all you Tom Cat groupies out there, don't panic. Our first statement is that we don't believe in marketing. The current fad is that marketing is not a dirty word. It's not. Our whole concept is based on establishing your core values and leadership. If you want to build your practice with Yellow Page ads, discounts, and coupons, don't read any further, and please consider throwing this book away.

Internal Marketing

We believe in internal promotion as the preferred form of marketing. Peter has referred to this in earlier chapters. In Thom's practice marketing means sending out all the reminders discussed earlier and occasionally a flier about a seminar series. Judi talks about community involvement in the chapter on ancillary services and that's a key point in any promotion effort. Building and educating your client base, participation in your community, and word of mouth will be far more effective than a coupon. Do we use value-added service? Yes! Do Peter's charts use the word *discount*? Yes. Did Thom use Ross Clark's Free Dental in his Las Vegas practice successfully? Yes. Let's not get lost in semantics.

If we develop a program to do multiple services in one visit, should we pass the savings on to our preferred clients? Of course; that's good business. In Thom's practice there is a special add-on service that includes an extra unit of anesthetic and dental cleaning and polishing with another surgical procedure. It is literally half the price of a Grade II dentistry. Is it good for the pet? Is it efficient for the practice? Is that internal marketing? Does the term *win–win* ring a bell?

Peter's current practice in rural northern Nevada doesn't celebrate national dental month, as his Las Vegas practice always did. In fact, there it was so successful, he did it twice a year! In Minden, with the add-on service, his techs have had to set limits on walk-in dentistry in the interest of good anesthetic protocols and late-night recovery. Some people would call that a discount. We'd call it good practice and excellent internal marketing.

Internal Promotion

If you follow Tom Cat's internal promotion programs, you know that staff training occurs two months before any promotion, then communication plans are built, and an outreach effort is initiated during the time between training and promotion. There is also an extended period following every promotion for preferred client access. Follow Judi's advice and write for a local paper, talk to the local schools, and speak at wives' clubs and local civic organizations at every opportunity. The communication portion of your annual marketing plan is an ongoing, continual program. Many high and middle schools have internship programs and career days. Are you represented? Involve your associates and nursing staff. They are still excited about their accomplishments and relish the chance to show off. Join local civic clubs before you tell them you are available to speak. Save some of those bladder stones, heartworm hearts, and other gross specimens for show-and-tell. Let your staff give tours on a regular basis. Hold an open house. After remodeling was done at Thom and Heather's hospital, their staff put together an awesome open house on a minimal budget. Stuffed animals were hooked up to all the doctors' toys (the fancy medical equipment). A staff member was in every room explaining its function and displaying x-rays, monitors, or models. The rest of the staff was conducting tours with practiced scripts so they wouldn't forget any important hospital functions. Other staff members brought in goodies from home. Everybody was impressed, the staff was proud, and the doctors did nothing but walk around with their mouths open! Whether in speaking, writing, or tours, educating your clients about available services or programs provides the necessary multiple exposures to establish and teach them about their pets' needs.

As discussed in detail earlier, word-of-mouth referrals from callbacks is astounding. We literally get referrals on a daily basis from clients who are impressed, not by our surgical and medical skill, but because we called them and asked about their pet. Then their neighbor comes in just to see a doctor who cares enough to call about a pet! Computer search and sorts and third-reminder callbacks give excellent internal monitors of the success of various programs and feedback on disasters. Better to learn of a problem firsthand than by community rumor mill! As mentioned earlier, *service is king*. Consider extended weekday hours, more weekend access, or even some form of emergency service. Depending on your geographical location, if you are the only clinic open at night, on weekends, or evening hours, word of mouth will spread your reputation like lightning. You certainly should use your newsletter, reminder cards, and invoices to announce the fact. You usually don't need expensive Yellow Page ads or advertising; military communities and those with high turnover may be an exception. The word will spread by the most important route, your satisfied clients! That's why one of our dozen dots is a chart on new clients with a subheading of new clients by referral. If you're not in a one-person practice or shareholder in the emergency clinic, consider taking emergencies. It's fun, lots of trauma, and one-on-one case management. It provides extra income for associates, either via ER fees and/or increased production, and clients love to go to their own doctor or hospital!

Teamwork

A sample marketing plan is provided in Figure 5.1. The fact is that it is a three-month plan per promotion. Of course you have to adapt it to your community, your geographical area, and your comfort level. The key to the three-month plan is that your staff training, your marketing, and your delivery have to be coordinated. Let's use national dental month as an example. If the doctors and technicians have been grading teeth all year long, you can do a search and sort to identify any grade II, III, or IV mouths that have not been taken care of in the last year. You could then bundle a program with a discount or a discounted nursing consultation to entice people into your practice during the slow month of February. You haven't gotten that far yet? Then the three-month program will get you started. We have a staff training meeting in December to stress the importance of dentistry, the side effects of periodontal disease, the importance of lab work to detect pre-existing disease, and all of our dental hygiene products. A doctors' meeting is required to calibrate our protocols, grading, and standard of care. All doctors and nurses must be consistent in order to support the staff and not confuse the clients. During the October/November budget meeting and again in January during budget review, we sit down with our inventory specialist to anticipate the increased product demand of each upcoming promotion. We also send out special notes on all the reminder cards and invoices each month to cross-sell upcoming promotions. We may even display all those free posters and client handouts left by our friendly distributors. Use only selected displays of targeted items rather than general meaningless billboards. A doctor or budding author in the practice may even create or rewrite a press release for an article for the local paper. All of these actions provide the 5-12 exposures necessary to establish the need in your client's mind explained below. Finally we make sure that the search and sort for dental reminders includes the entire past year. Now we're ready for the special in February. This concept applies to the entire marketing plan in Figure 5.1. Whether it's x-ray awareness to remind our doctors of our standard of care, parasite prevention, or allergy and arthritis

SAMPLE MARKETING PLAN

Month	Training	Marketing	Service
December	Dental	Senior's newsletter	Wellness exam for holiday puppies
January	Heartworm	Dental	Lead II ECG screening
February	Internal parasites	Heartworm	Dental month
March	External parasites	Internal parasites	Heartworm clinic
April	IV catheters, parvo testing	External parasites	2 for 1 fecals
May	Vaccine & wellness protocols	Parvo awareness	Flea & tick baths
June	Outpatient nurse, TPR, dental grading	Boarding tips and wellness newsletter	Parvo season
July	Nutritional counseling	Tech exams, preferred client	Boarding season
August	X-ray & arthritis screening	Jenny Craig month	Busy time & staff vacation
September	Chocolate, tinsel, and other toxins	Prepare for fall slow down	Free weigh-ins and counseling
October	Pet placement	Holiday Newsletter	Arthritis screening program
November	Cardiac awareness	Don't buy a surprise	Caution for holidays pet handout!

FIGURE 5.1

screening months, training is followed by marketing.

Both must precede any successful program. Regular doctor meetings followed by staff training set the precedent for successful marketing. No matter how much you think you are aware, none of us can talk about parasites, skin care, behavior, medicine, surgery, genetic screening, planned parenthood, nutrition, boarding, vaccinations, current controversies, over-the-counter items, ancillary services, dentistry, current physical examination findings, baseline wellness items and laboratory tests, and (get the picture) on every visit. Even a great nursing and reception staff cannot do it every time! It is necessary for staff and doctors alike to recycle training and awareness programs. In fact it's necessary to remind our clients of these issues periodically as well.

Persuasion Rather Than Selling

We have said the key promotion words before:

The only thing a veterinary practice ever sells consistently is peace of mind.

We clearly state needs (not make recommendations), then become silent and listen.

The client is allowed to buy from two yes options.

The closure question is always, "Is this the level of care you want today?"

The New American Veterinary Practice

In promotions for tomorrow's clients, a practice must understand the ways of change—the paradigm shifts—of the new millennium, including:

Not cost containment—rather—increased productivity

Not staff recruitment and training—rather—staff retention and recognition

Not pennies per CWT cures—rather—patient advocacy for wellness

Not guest relations—rather—client-centered service and system improvement

Not within the job description—rather—exceeding job expectations

Not a mission statement—rather—core values with a mission focus

Not responding to competition—rather—meeting unmet needs

Not just gross income increases—rather—programs that drive more net!

Vendors usually build great brochures for the client, and sometimes monographs for the doctors, but who builds the marketing piece for the staff? Who helps the staff and young associate doctors become patient advocates, while sharing products and services? This is what we call in-service training requirements, which are based on the Ten New Marketing Rules for the New Millennium:

1. Change the rules—redefine, break habits, and alter restraining factors (paradigms).
2. Develop strategic foresight—watch community trends, acknowledge the community changes, respond to emerging community needs.
3. Innovate—create new services, retool tired programs, invent new nomenclature, implement over 60 percent of all new staff ideas within 48 hours.
4. Time your actions—to external growth, internal effectiveness, long-range plans.
5. Think and act quickly—capture the moment, form a strategic response, pursue rapid implementation.
6. Customize your services—know your target audience, provide definite variations to client demands, accept the diversity of client desires as reality.
7. Restructure—add inventory teams, outpatient nurses, behavior management counselors, and other paraprofessional veterinary extenders.
8. Manage diversity—more fully utilize the female staff, ethnic diversity, generation X, and other staff decision makers on your team.
9. Empower your people—encourage intellectual energy, reward commitment, promote non-linear thinking (e.g., mind-map brainstorming).
10. Continue to learn—promote organizational adaptation, pursue continual job redesign, develop system thinking.

The companion animal veterinary practice of the new millennium must respond to the client's perceived needs, which means:

✓ talking in their terminology,
✓ getting them in and out quickly, and
✓ speaking for the patient in a caring and concerned manner.

This "tuning in to the perceived needs" means having Internet awareness, scientific astuteness, and a community focus. It means learning to give two "yes" options (>75% acceptance rate) to meet each patient's need(s), never entering a "yes versus no" situation (<50% acceptance rate). The ONLY thing a veterinary healthcare professional "sells" is peace of mind; all else the client is allowed to buy from the two "yes" options of wellness or curative care. The outpatient nursing staff, client relations (front) team, and doctors must therefore:

- Know what the emerging community trends are.
- Offer current literature to address the community's pet needs.
- Show how industry has developed the product/service to meet the needs.
- Offer a care-based model that allows the staff to help the client & patient.
- Meet the price concerns with a participative net projection staff scenario.
- Ensure that the staff understands their role in patient advocacy with the products.

The Five P's of Marketing

The Five P's of marketing are PRODUCT, PRICE, PLACE, PROMOTION, and PROGRAMS; the terms are self-explanatory. The old sales approach used by many was to pursue selling by AIDA:

✓ Get the person's Attention.
✓ Develop their Interest.
✓ Stimulate their Desire.
✓ Force some kind of Action.

Today, the progressive and tuned-in sales systems are shifting to a persuasion method, with both a "Seller's Persuasion Process" and a "Buyer's Process" of thought and action planning. The persuasion skills are not simple or easy to acquire; they are frightfully complicated. The awareness can be facilitated, as can the plan, but you MUST focus on the human behavior within the specific veterinary practice; this is a major variable!

The Seller's Persuasion Process has five parts:

✓ Needs (seller's awareness of veterinary population)
✓ Plan (addressing the practice's needs—patient advocacy)

✓ How it works (outline for buy-in of plan)
✓ Results (payoff to the practice)
✓ Next step (commitment to buy within time frame available)

There are five parts of the buying process:

✓ The process begins when there is an **unsatisfied need.** No one does anything without a need. It supplies the motivation. It is a need as seen by the buyer, not the seller. It is as they see it, feel it, or just know it. It may be real or imagined, concrete or abstract, rational or irrational, but a need must be there!
✓ The mere presence of a need is not enough to stimulate action. It must be **sufficiently important** to raise the priority for immediate attention. Recognition of the need as something that must be filled is step two.
✓ The active part of the buying mode is **the search.** This is as quick and easy as a purchase from a trusted distributor, or maybe just the best price if there is no knowledge about quality.
✓ **Evaluation** is the assessment of search data. Anyone can "low bid" a due out. The search findings are compared to the needs list, and options begin to appear.
✓ The **decision to take a specific action** is based on positive information. If the data is not positive, a "buy" decision may not be made.

What really happens in persuasion marketing is an alignment of the seller's process to the buyer's needs:

FIGURE 5.2

```
┌───────────────────────────────────────────────────┐
│                                                     │
│        COMMIT THIS CHART TO MEMORY                  │
│                                                     │
│     Buyer's Process              Seller's Process   │
│                                                     │
│        Needs           ⇦           Needs            │
│                                                     │
│        Recognition     ⇦           Plan             │
│                                                     │
│        Search          ⇦           How It Works     │
│                                                     │
│        Evaluation      ⇦           Results          │
│                                                     │
│        Decision        ⇦           Next Stop        │
│                                                     │
└───────────────────────────────────────────────────┘
```

Persuasion Marketing—Relationship between Buyer and Seller

Most buying decisions are made based on feelings. In the absence of knowledge or feelings, the decision is usually made based on the economics. Most all people have only a finite amount of money to spend, so the mass marketing specialists attempt to change feelings by elevating their product's importance by repetition, sometimes with a color or sound associated so the senses are concurrently excited. This causes feelings to be developed in the potential customers. The same thing happens with clients of veterinary practices, and it is accentuated by the fact that clients are already coming into the practice stressed. They are usually concerned about the animal's health, about the threat of disease, or more often, about the cost of restoring or protecting the wellness of their animal.

The popular spectrum of feelings was first described in modern literature in the early 1940s in a thesis by Abraham Maslow entitled the "Hierarchy of Needs." He used a triangle to describe the human needs, from the most basic foundation needs (physiological: housing, food, clothing, etc.) to the most rewarding (self-actualization). He described the critical nature of human response, the re-

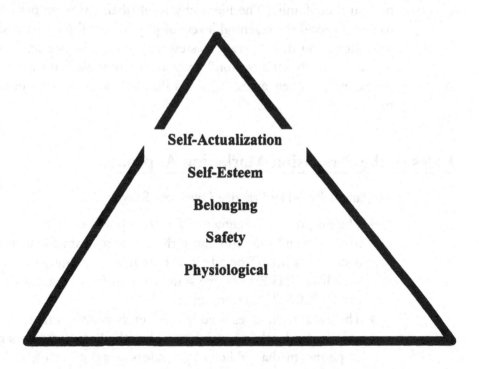

FIGURE 5.3

Maslow's Hierarchy of Needs Triangle

quirement to meet all basic needs before a person can "ascend" the hierarchy of needs to the next level. He also stated that someone can have multiple "hierarchy triangles" going concurrently in their life.

Part of Maslow's original thesis was a disclaimer, "Don't believe it is this simple; it is for discussion of the theory only!" which has been ignored over the last half century by most people using the "triangle" to discuss marketing (and other human responses). Maslow's triangle only provides a model for discussion, because in real life, due to environmental conditions, someone can be at multiple levels in various aspects of their life at a single point in time, depending on which life or operational aspect is being evaluated at that moment (e.g., consider the multiple roles of a single individual who is a mother, veterinarian, church elder, Rotary member, wife, double black diamond skier, and child to an ailing parent).

This disclaimer concept aside, most people who have accepted stewardship of their family pet also consider that animal to be a member of their family. About one-third of those give their pet "people status" in their family. The hierarchy level of the average pet owner is usually beyond the essential levels of physiological security and physical safety, and they operate as stewards in the "belonging," "self-esteem," or "self-actualization" areas of the triangle. This is an important concept when assessing the value and approach of persuasion marketing.

Rules of the Persuasion Marketing Approach

Alignment #1—The Practice Overview Survey

- ♦ The purpose of Alignment #1 is to define the "seller's" objective into a "plan" that will cause the buyer to want the next step to occur. This MUST be a logical flow from beginning to end, using the OBJECTIVE to derive statements of PLAN, and also to feed the NEXT STEP commitment.
- ♦ The usual techniques used by veterinary practices that are applicable to this level are: newsletters, health alerts, reminders by mail or phone, media publicity by vendors or associations, and similar "informational" exposures.

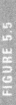

ALIGNMENT #1
_____

Objective Driven
- Goals & Commitment
    - ✓ Core Values
    - ✓ Vision
- Awareness of Needs of Client
    - ✓ Community Trends
    - ✓ Product Trends
    - ✓ Patient Advocacy
- Jointly Planning the Next Step
_____

Alignment #2—The professional's ability to meet the needs

♦ The NEEDS of the client and patient should be completely developed, and the RESULTS should translate the NEEDS into appropriate patient and client BENEFITS. This sequence is critical.

♦ The usual techniques used by veterinary practices that are applicable to this level are: receptionist awareness, outpatient nurse contact, and eventually doctor statements of need.

ALIGNMENT #2
_____

Responding to the Client's Perceptions
- Awareness of Practice Needs
- Plan the Practice Sequence
    - ✓ Speak to the Pet's Needs
    - ✓ Reduced Cost by Adding Value
- Potential Payoff Benefit's to Client
    - ✓ Peace of Mind
    - ✓ Alternatives & Options
    - ✓ Fulfull Existing Perceived Need
_____

Alignment #3—The "Prescription" Time, adding product, promotion, and price to place

♦ Alignment #3 is HOW IT WORKS. At this time, you should tell the clients only what they need to know in principle to understand how the PLAN will be carried out. Do not overburden them with theory at this final phase.

♦ The usual techniques used by veterinary practices that are applicable to this level are: the "two yes" options, setting priorities for healthcare delivery, establishing the next contact expectation, and describing the consequence(s) of no action.

FIGURE 5.6

ALIGNMENT #3

Sell Peace of Mind ⟶ Let Them Buy
- Practice's Need for Action
    - ✓ Treatment/care of Choice
    - ✓ Sense of Urgency
- How It Works
    - ✓ Outline of Buy-In (not details)
    - ✓ Pay-Off for Client
    - ✓ Patient Benefit
- Commitment to Buy
    - ✓ Within Set Time
    - ✓ Next Visit Commitment

With the three alignments of persuasion marketing in mind, the relationships in the sequence can be placed into a single table for ease of understanding. These relationships illustrate and review the five parts of the buying process and compare them to the five parts of the selling process:

FIGURE 5.7

STRUCTURE AND ALIGNMENTS CHART

Structure	Alignments		
Audience	(1)	(2)	(3)
Objective	OBJECTIVE		
Needs	↕	NEEDS	
Plan	Plan	↕	PLAN ↕
HIW	↕	↕	HIW
Results	↕	RESULTS	
Next Step	NEXT STEP		

Chapter Five of Volume 2 discusses the means of differentiating yourself within your demographic, geographic, and psychographic community. In this book we are focusing on the development of programs within your practice that people can choose from. This approach unto itself will differentiate a practice from its colleagues in the neighborhood. If one aspect of marketing is to give clients what they need or want, isn't giving them a choice a form of marketing?

How do we best market these programs to our clients? We have always felt that marketing is an education process and/or a problem-solving process. Any time we develop a marketing plan, we seek acceptance by education. It took a long time for people to accept that their pets had teeth that needed care.

First, people had to be educated that dental disease existed in dogs and cats.

Second, people had to be taught that dental disease is both painful and dangerous.

Third, people had to be informed that we (the veterinarians) could solve this problem.

This education process was necessary not only for the clients but also for the veterinarians and their staff. Now, we have clients coming in and telling us that their pets need their teeth cleaned. Having taught the clients this well, we now need to reward their actions by encouraging them and making early and proactive dental care more affordable. Isn't this an example of marketing by education and information exchange?

Thus, let's consider marketing a form of education and persuasion. When developing a marketing plan, we must:

1. Educate ourselves.
2. Educate our paraprofessionals.
3. Educate our clients.

Educating Ourselves

Before we can comfortably and confidently present a new product or service to our staff, we must believe in it ourselves. Whether it's a new or recently released pharmaceutical or a new surgical technique, a new diet or an old philosophy, we must have read and researched or investigated it completely.

From manufacturers to distributors, Internet to mail, we should read and learn as much as necessary on the issue to have a comfort zone. We must believe in and understand the level of care that we are going to market and the problems that we are going to solve for our patients and their owners.

Education of Our Paraprofessionals

This very much parallels the research we did for ourselves. It may also include lunch meetings by manufacturers, videotapes, or training CDs. Role playing as a teaching modality cannot be overemphasized. The final outcome is that the staff must understand and believe in your practice programs.

Educating Our Clients

Veterinarians are problem solvers. We meet the needs of our patients. Thus we must educate the clients on the problems that their pets have. Knowledge of each problem and a complete understanding of the ramifications of failing to deal with the problem are what we must provide to our clients. Then, without much effort, clients will be willing to fulfill their pets' needs.

Handouts, brochures, videotapes, and information on hold are just a few examples of tools of the trade. Let's use an example.

Pain Management—An Example of Education-Led Marketing

Thinking back to veterinary school, I can recall a discussion of pain receptors and pain in the pharmacology class and possibly during the anesthesia class and rotation. Pain management seemed to be reserved for orthopedic procedures and/or intervertebral disk disease cases.

For the first few years out of school, pain management consisted of aspirin, corticosteroids, and maybe a little butorphanol, but rarely anything else. I remember hearing myself say, "Dogs and cats have much higher pain thresholds than we do." "We tend to avoid pain management because the pain acts as a means of keeping the pets quieter as they recover from surgery." "We don't have a lot of pain management drugs because narcotics are so difficult to control and dangerous to have around the staff, and people might break in and steal them." I look back now on these statements and laugh.

I don't recall when pain management became vogue. I remember a Fort Dodge salesperson talking about mixing Torbutrol with V.A.L. syrup for use post-declaws and post-extractions. I remember attending some continuing education sessions in Las Vegas on surgery and anesthesia and hearing about "the patch." I read numerous articles in the journals that slowly over time introduced me to the truth in pain control: It hurts animals just as much as it hurts us. So, obviously, the drug companies did their job selling the concept of pain control to me.

Having bought into the need for pain control, I started to become more and more interested in how it could become an integral part of our quality care program. Suddenly, narcotics didn't seem so outlandish. Rimadyl and Etogesic opened up new pain control pathways and "the patch" was not Nicoderm but Fentanyl. As I saw more, heard more, and read more, I started to experiment more in the clinic. All declaws got Torbutrol injections pre-operatively. Extractions went home with Torbutrol syrup. More and more aspirin was used. Then Rimadyl. Any major exploratory or orthopedic was patched. And I started to include pain management in the estimates I gave. Fewer and fewer animals recovered screaming or refusing to move or eat for 24 to 72 hours. The staff was intrigued. I was sold. Now I needed to teach the staff.

Teaching the staff was no problem. They all experience pain. Whether it's a migraine or a dog bite, pain is an aspect of everyday life in a practice. The staff was going through 500 acetaminophen per month; they could very easily accept the need for pain control on our patients. We discussed the different types—narcotic, nonsteroidal anti-inflammatory, etc. The declaws recovered much more smoothly when drugs were on board. They were happy, I was happy. Soon the clients would understand and be happy, too.

Initially, pain management was an option presented to the client upon admission for a procedure. The staff talked about how anesthesia provides a small, short-term analgesia peri-operatively, but we could offer more pain control, at a price. Clients who had had pets for years said, "All my other pets did OK without it." New pet owners and people who had suffered themselves questioned why we had to charge for it. "Shouldn't it be part of the surgery and anesthesia cost, what do you mean you don't routinely include pain management?" Soon, we took the decision-making process out of the hands of clients and included minor pain management costs in the prices quoted for all minor electives. We offered upgraded pain management for those cases deemed appropriate. Now, pain management isn't an issue or question. Clients recognize that the last thing that they want is for their pet to feel any untoward pain. They routinely ask for additional pain control even for routine dental care without extractions, declaws, etc. We educated our clients in the exam room, via newsletters, and just by open frank discussion. Now, they ask for it.

Create a separate revenue category for pain management and start to track your revenues for pain management alone. You will be amazed.

The philosophy behind this is that you, the doctor or manager, are sold on the pet's need for something. You develop a complete understanding of the product or service. You educate the staff on the importance of the service or procedure. They buy into it. Finally, you introduce your clients to it, slowly at first, and then more rapidly.

The most successful marketing program is one where, with minimal exposure, a client requests a service without prompting. Now, see one, do one, teach one. Or sell one.

Are you confused or do you see a pattern here? We started the chapter with one clinician's options. In the middle we gave you some new theories about sales and marketing. At the end we went back to another clinician's option or perspective or approach. The real key is to reread the chapter and look for the common elements to make your own plan.

    ✓ Identify the *need* for your client and pet.
    ✓ Educate your staff of the *need* with a *program*.
    ✓ *Promote* the *program* to satisfy the *need*.

Kind of like the SOAP we're used to.

Ancillary Services 6

Moneymaking opportunities that do not require an extended education abound in veterinary medicine. They require a creative, active imagination. Veterinary hospital, resort, grooming, boutique, and nutrition center are all part of the one-stop shopping theory for your client's pets.

The construction of a boarding facility expansion may cost only half as much as a hospital costs, if planned with pigmented concrete floors, simple construction hog panel dividers, and easy-to-clean surfaces. One pet partner can attend to 33 guests in an eight-hour shift. Some skilled managers, or heavy cat populations, can increase this to 48 guests. Self-watering systems and central disinfectant dispensers with quick release hoses for cleaning decrease cleaning time. Industrial quality washers and dryers save time and maintenance costs. The third edition of Tom Cat's AAHA Design Starter Kit for Veterinary Hospitals includes a boarding section. This is one area where a skilled team of consultants can really help a practice's expansion project.

Pet Resort

A high net income will be realized with a properly managed boarding operation. A shift in nomenclature is essential to convey to the public the quality facility and services you have to offer. By adopting this stance, your attitude is contagious to the staff, and the attitude of the staff will spill over onto your clientele. Remember, this playful approach is for the kennel (resort) areas only and is not recommended for your hospital. Here are some examples:

- Boarding Kennel becomes Pet Resort
- Boarding Animal becomes Resort Guest

- Kennel Worker becomes Pet Partner
- Exercise Yard becomes Courtyard, Playground, or Pet Park
- Dog Run becomes Guest Room
- Cat Cage becomes Cat Condo Units
- "We feed in the morning" becomes "Breakfast is served between 7 and 8"

It is imperative that the dog and cat boarding areas be impeccably clean and odor free. Cats and dogs should not be maintained in the same room. The old philosophy of keeping different species in the same room to dilute disease does not have any place here due to the simple fact that pets with diseases should not be kept in your resort areas at all.

Factors such as front drains vs. rear drains, automatic flush systems vs. manual flush systems or the manufacturer of your cat condos are personal preferences. Factors such as odor control, adequate air exchange, light, sanitation, and noise control allow for no choices. They absolutely have to be present for quality. Odor control, proper air exchange, and sanitation can be linked together. You cannot have one without the other. Overlighting your resort areas requires a totally clean area and has a positive effect on your guests. A mix of natural lighting with water-resistant artificial lighting is recommended. Sound baffles should be used for noise absorption. A more detailed description of building materials, engineering, and design are not within the scope of this chapter.

The majority of pet owners will have made an appointment before leaving their pet (family member). At the time an appointment is made, or at least at the time of admission, retrieve information on where the owner can be reached, discharge date and time, feeding preferences, vaccination history, medications to be given, a list of the pet's personal belongings left at the resort, and any other pertinent information. Remind clients of special packages that the resort may provide. Many owners are leaving their pets to go on vacation, and their guilt is lessened if they know their pet is having a vacation as well. These extra services equal extra net income. Acquiring the information prior to the time of admission will save the client time on the day of check-in and will help prevent confusion. Your resort instills a sense of security in the owner of a caring and safe environment by showing attention to detail. See Figure 6.1 for a sample check-in card that doubles as a report card.

FIGURE 6.1

Report Card

Owner's Name

Pet's Name _____ Apt Number _____

Breed _____ Age _____ Sex _____ Diet _____ Weight _____

Special VIP Packages _____ Luggage _____

Comments

Day	1	2	3	4	5-6	7	8	9	10	11	12	13	14	15	16	17	18	19	20	21	22	23	24	25	26	27	28	29	30
Stool																													
Urine																													
AM meal																													
PM meal																													
Special Diet																													
Personality																													
Appearance																													

Explanation

Stool: 1 Normal
2 None
3 Soft
4 Diarrhea
5 Worms
6 Blood/Mucous

Urine: 1 Normal
2 None
3 Blood

Meals: 1 Ate All
2 Ate Some
3 Not hungry

Personality: 1 Active
2 Good
3 Fair
4 depressed

Appearance: 1 Happy
2 Fair
3 Homesick

Please: Check Your Pet's Luggage

A large percentage of owners will want to tour the facility. Touring is excellent public relations and should be welcomed. Make sure the pet partners understand this and perceive these tours as an opportunity to convey pride in their job as well as in the resort. Offer a tour at the time the reservation is made. Many clients will feel more comfortable with the resort after this offer, even if they don't actually take you up on the tour. Just knowing you have nothing to hide makes them feel better.

Create a detailed resort policy that includes all services, hours of operation, vaccination requirements, and fees. Make sure all clients receive a resort policy and have documentation of its receipt in their records. This documentation can prevent later conflicts over, for example, fees and time of discharge. This should be inexpensive and reproducible in-house due to the high likelihood for changes and additions.

The resort brochure should be a separate source of information. It will remain fairly constant and is best if professionally prepared. Use these brochures for mailings as well as for handouts to clients. Some professional groups will include information on your resort in their contacts with newcomers to town. This can be somewhat expensive. Other alternatives include using credit reports to look for changes in addresses. The electric company will also usually allow you to check addresses with new service hookups. Be resourceful. Make sending a brochure with a welcome letter to newcomers part of your monthly marketing strategy. Offer to send a brochure and resort policy to all clients when they make a reservation or just call to inquire about the resort.

Allow for extensive training time with your resort staff so that any indication of pet illness can be detected early. Proper training cannot be emphasized enough. Guests should have a checks-over by a pet partner prior to being placed in their guest rooms. If possible, do this brief exam with the owner present. By doing so, the owner witnesses the complimentary exam, thereby setting the tone for the level of care that their pet will receive during its stay. It also allows for any abnormalities and recommended solutions to be discussed. Remarks such as, "My pet couldn't possibly have fleas unless she got them here," can be thwarted.

Ten Tips for a Successful Resort Operation

1. Employ only quality, caring pet partners. Pay good wages to hire good employees. The number of details each pet partner must remember is tremendous and requires desire and intelligence.
2. Consider the resort staff equal to the hospital staff. Do not allow separations in importance to occur.
3. All guests must have a neck band and a cage card that lists important information. This is mandatory to prevent errors. Enforce the rule that the last task performed before leaving for the day is to do a walk-through to check on each and every guest and to give them a bedtime snack (dog biscuit) as we walk through. We call this "tucking them in."
4. If the owner brings food from home for their pet, be sure to feed it. When it is not used, some owners believe their pet was not fed anything during its stay, or at the least did not eat the diet offered.
5. White boards are necessities.

    Use a white board in a main traffic area to display the location of each guest. Guest rooms should be numbered and coincide with the number on the diagram displayed on the white board. Assign a pet partner to update the board as needed during the day.

    Use a white board to indicate which guest is receiving special packages. It is also important to document in the boarding chart what specials are to be provided; then date and check off in the record that they have been done.

    Use a white board to indicate which guests are to go home each day with the estimated time of pickup. One pet partner should be in charge of doing this as their first task each morning. It will aid the entire staff in doing their specific jobs in a timely manner.

WHITE BOARD FOR RESORT

Guest's name	Last name	Room number	Special packages	Medication	Special diet
Cricket	Haig	1	playtime	heartworm	Sci Maint
Schnaps	Howell	2	brush and run	thyroid bid	K/D
Skylar	Dempsey	3	none	none	lames
Augie	Webster	4	hike	ears	R/D

FIGURE 6.2

6. Offer a complimentary cleansing bath to all dogs staying over two nights. Bathe cats at the owner's request only and for an additional fee, but do brush each cat on the day of discharge. A cat's natural shedding ability is hindered when it has little to rub against; therefore, the owner may perceive the excessive shedding as neglect by the resort. The resort will receive many complements when the guests go home cleaner and better groomed than when they came. Explain to the owner that bathing and drying requires care and cannot be rushed. Designate a time when these guests can be picked up to prevent owner waiting and frustration.

7. Set your policy concerning dropped off toys and bedding. If you are going to pamper your guests and their owners, using their personal belongings will be a necessity. Plan ahead to deal with the associated problems. Require that all bedding and toys be marked with the client's last name in permanent ink. Bedding can also be marked or tagged with a dry cleaning tag that won't be removed by laundering. Toys should be listed on the guest's arrival card or cage card. Hanging baskets on the doors of suites can also be used to keep track of multiple toys.

8. VIP Packages should be offered and discussed with each new guest owner. These packages will vary from one extra service to a group of extra services. Document in the record which package was chosen so that you will be knowledgeable about the clients' desires for their pet upon return visits. Again here is a chance to use your imagination and practice your marketing skills. These extras are another way to set your resort above the others in your area.

9. Have a pet partner phone the owner the day after discharge to check up on the pet, to ask how they perceived their stay, and to remind the owner that the entire resort staff is there should they need anything. Always refer to the pet by name and document this phone call in the record with the date, comment from owner, and initials of the pet partner making the phone call.

10. As the owner of the resort, make certain that you walk through the facility daily. This allows you to see that your expectations are being met, and it also makes you accessible, if only briefly, to the resort staff. This is very important.

Image

- Portray an interesting visual image throughout all high traffic areas of facility. Decorate with fun, inexpensive artwork, e.g., funny pet cartoons blown up and framed.
- Provide *current* magazines. Subscribe to several that appeal to your diverse clients. Don't forget the children.
- Provide a daily newspaper. Assign one employee to scan the local paper for articles about clients and mail them with message of "Glad you made the news."
- Keep reception desk neat and noncluttered.
- Have staff wear clean, neat coordinating uniforms.
- Provide all staff members with name tags.

Consider giving a clever, individual name to your resort that will give it an identity separate from your hospital. This will allow for creative advertising and marketing that may not coincide with your strategies concerning your hospital. One excellent method for advertising is a pickup and delivery service. A modified cargo van with individual cubicles is ideal. Consider having Dalmatian spots and the title "Resort Limousine" designed and painted or applied to the outside. Most practices have a utility vehicle, so take advantage of any opportunity to market. A mileage log must be kept for tax purposes. The log also gives a check to be certain all trips are charged out to the client. Because this service is performed outside of the facility, it seems to be a fee that is easily overlooked. Make sure your fee for this service is in sync with its importance. When calculating fees, consider cost of vehicle, insurance, gasoline, maintenance, tag and taxes, and the employee's time.

Extra Services

Extra services that may be offered include playtime, walks, special pampering, bedtime stories, brush and run, medicated boarding, and any others you can think up. Be creative. Have a staff brainstorming session. What additional services would you want for your pet if you were leaving him or her at a resort? These services can then be bundled into packages or offered separately. When an owner purchases extra services, make sure your pet partners document with initials, date, and time each time they perform those services.

See Figures 6.1 and 6.3 for report cards on special services. When the guest is discharged, tell the owner, "Fifi really enjoyed her daily game of Frisbee." Make some comment to ensure that the owners know the services were given and give them a report card to take home.

Here are some other ideas to attract attention to your service:

- K-9 courtyard with multiple play areas. It should be fenced with good visibility to the public. Pea gravel makes a good ground cover. Keep clean! Pick up 2–3 times daily.
- VIP boarding. Includes playtime, daily brushing, fleece blanket, treats, and complimentary weekly baths
- Cattery. Soundproof, include exercise area, aquarium

Pet Sitting

- Extend boarding services to include pet sitting at a client's home.
- Fees are determined by the extent of services and distance traveled. If an employee works after or before hours, pay by percentage.
- Check with the owner on the necessity of becoming bonded.

Advertising

Mainstream Advertising

One suggestion for advertising is to compose serial advertisements for the local newspaper using faux testimonials from your guests (not clients). See Appendix 4 for sample testimonials and other resort forms. A great pat on the back for your groomers and pet partners is to include them in your overall marketing and advertising plan.

Newspaper Article

Write a weekly column for your local newspaper. Becoming a contributing columnist may require work, but the rewards from the exposure are priceless. Contact the editor of the newspaper with your idea, prepared to show examples. If your idea is rejected at first, expect it, and try again in one to two months armed with more example articles. Do not give up easily.

A question-and-answer format is pleasing to the public. The ques-

FIGURE 6.3

Medication Record for Boarding Guest

_____

Medication(s)_____

_____

Instructions_____

_____

_____

Date	Morning	Pet Partner	Noon	Pet Partner	Night	Pet Partner
1						
2						
3						
4						
5						
6						
7						
8						
9						
10						
11						
12						
13						
14						
15						
16						
17						
18						
19						
20						
21						
22						
23						
24						
25						
26						
27						
28						
29						
30						

tions asked of you each week in the consultation room are an endless source of material if you do not have any actual mailed-in questions to choose from. In the public's mind, having a column in the newspaper makes you the authority in the community.

Special Events

The possibilities for special events are endless. This is an excellent opportunity to involve the entire staff, not merely for implementation, but, more importantly, for creation. Schedule an annual brainstorming session centered around lunch, dessert, or some type of social activity. To plan for special events—social events with marketing overtones—you and your staff need to be in a social mood. This meeting should be one that is looked forward to by you and your staff.

An example of a festive event is to offer complimentary photographs with Santa Dog. Pick a Saturday at the beginning of December for the event to occur. Begin running advertisements in the local newspaper a week or so ahead. The newspaper's ad department will help with the design at no additional charge if needed. Make an effort to recruit an amateur photographer, thereby minimizing expenses. Photography and animals seem to go together, so this task should not be too difficult. Next consider Santa's costume. A good Santa suit is easy to find, although locating the ideal dog head (or whatever animal you choose) may require some investigating, so plan ahead. Initially renting the costume is the best idea, but if this becomes an annual event it will be more economical in most cases to purchase one. Other costume considerations are elf suits for the staff. Get everyone involved with a high level of enthusiasm, and this annual event will become greatly anticipated by the community.

Make certain that Santa is trained in animal handling. Some dogs sit perfectly still, whereas some cats want to perch on top of Santa's head, and a snake or two will try to wrap around and become Santa's belt. Dropping a ferret and seeing it bounce across the room followed by two Labradors is not amusing to the owner.

Plan ahead such things as film purchase, what snacks to be served, the location and composition of the photo shoot, and the flow of traffic. Compose a sign-in sheet with a numerical system that corresponds with the roll of film being shot. This helps decrease confusion when the owner returns for the photos. Some owners will want the negatives. This policy will need to be discussed and determined with the photographer. Have a system worked out for photo pickup days. You do not want 100+ people coming in on the same day. This can be implemented into the sign up sheet and conveyed to the owner at the time of check-in.

Make the event open to the public, not exclusive to your established clients. If you have animals boarding, be sure to photograph them during slow times. Also include the appropriate hospitalized pets. The more animals you photograph the more word-of-mouth publicity you receive, and of course, the more successful your event will be. Do not let the event interfere with the regular daily operations of appointments, emergencies, etc.

Another marketing idea is doggie field trips. While your pet partners are exercising guests, have them take pictures of the hike they took or the game of catch they played. Give these to the owner at discharge with a note from the guest about how much they enjoyed their stay. At Thanksgiving or Halloween put together goodie bags of leftovers or "trick or treats" that their pet received. These can be biscuits or catnip toys. During holiday periods, send guests home wearing festive holiday print bandanas. You can make these inexpensively using fabric purchased at the local fabric store and crimping scissors.

Community Involvement

The saying from Chapter One, "the door must swing," aptly describes the underpinnings of business success. To make this happen, market yourself, your greatest commodity. Do not stand behind your exam or surgery tables and expect clients to swing your front door in great anticipation of meeting you—they won't! Go out into the community and meet your current and potential clients. Here are a few ideas:

Join a civic club and be more than a member occupying a seat at lunch once a week. Be active!

Support the Chamber of Commerce or Community Development Foundation. This is an excellent way to make business contacts and simultaneously demonstrate that you and your business support the community.

If it is in line with your theology, join a local church.

Make appointments with local principals or others at schools in charge of guest speakers. Make known your availability and enthusiasm to speak to the students about veterinary medicine. Market the availability of your facility for guided tours.

Meet with area scouting directors and do the same as with the school administrators. Sponsor an Explorer Scouting Post.

Sponsor a youth sport team when this is part of the city parks and recreation program for your area. Having 20-plus children wearing a T-shirt with your business' name on it for several hours each week with parents, grandparents, and friends present is community involvement doubling as good advertising. Have the T-shirts printed with a logo that will get noticed.

Display locally produced artwork on a wall in your waiting room. Artists and animals often go hand in hand. Cater to artwork from area schools as well as to the adult artist sector.

Community involvement must also include social activities. Attend area ballet and symphony performances as well as theater productions.

Support local charities such as the United Way. You may advertise a United Way Day and donate a percentage of your gross for that day.

Marketing yourself may feel unnatural at first, but especially in the early stages of your business it needs to be done. See and be seen. Set the example, expect and direct a degree of community involvement from your staff as well, and "watch the door swing!"

Grooming

Grooming is a necessary service to include in your facility. Who would like to go to a resort that did not provide a spa? The more services you offer—hospital, resort, grooming, nutrition, boutique—the more pet owners bring you to mind and the more often they come in. All this spells profit.

You may hire groomers as independent contractors where they lease space you provide in your facility. The groomers run it as a separate business with their own staff. They set and collect their own fees, but your pet partners refer business to them. Negotiate a discount for resort guests staying a certain period of time as part of the lease. If the pet is moved to the grooming area, you provide the incentive of no charge for boarding on the last day.

A second method of employment pays the groomer on commission. Percentages for commission vary, but they usually lie within the ranges of 50 percent owner:50 percent groomer to 40 percent owner:60 percent groomer. When you find an accomplished groomer with a positive attitude, offer them benefits that make them want to stay and be a part of the team. A good groomer is a very valuable asset. There are many legal issues to be researched before you categorize a groomer under contract labor. These should be carefully considered to prevent any repercussions by the IRS.

It is best to have groomers working under contract. Contracts identify expectations and help avoid controversies.

Your pet partners should routinely do the cleansing baths for resort guests. It is not economical to pay the groomer for these baths when the hourly employees have this in their job description. Reinforce this procedure with the groomers and the pet partners so that they all work well together as a team. Explain that all days are different, and on any given day they may need to modify this plan. Grooming, bathing, drying, and brushing pets is time consuming when done correctly. I cannot emphasize enough the need for the grooming staff and the resort staff to understand that they are part of the same team.

The groomer should be available to admit all new grooming guests, and consult with the owner on exactly what type of clip they want for their pet. This should be documented in the grooming chart. On subsequent visits, if the same style is desired, it is not critical for the groomer to be on hand at the time of admission, but remember, the more contact the groomer has with the owner, the greater the bonding. Have the groomer recommend when the pet will need its next haircut and set it up before the client leaves. To lessen missed appointments a confirming phone call should be made the day prior to the pet's salon day. A banner way to convey your resort's caring attitude is to phone the client the next day to check on how the pet is enjoying its new coif.

Pet Boutique

An upscale Pet Boutique is a profit center. All that needs to be done apart from maintaining a reasonable inventory is to offer good quality merchandise. No appointments, no office visits, no surgery! Easy!

Purchase upper-end products to avoid competition with the large retail stores—since you can't. Once again, use your imagination! Commission a local leather worker to make leather leashes, collars, and harnesses. Contact a seamstress to design and make original fleece sweaters. Coordinate with ceramists to create art with animal themes. The possibilities are endless. Do not settle for mediocrity. These items may be expensive, but they are available exclusively at your boutique, and a guarantee should accompany every sale.

Pet Nutrition Center

Do you have a pet nutrition center or dog food in a back room? Do you have nutrition counselors or kids carrying food? This area may be part of the boutique, resort, or hospital. You may have two areas—one for premium diets in the resort and a separate area for prescription products in the hospital.

Some resorts and hospitals have large point of purchase displays. These are often provided or paid for by food companies. Other hospitals and resorts display only cans or small bags in exam or waiting areas to stimulate discussion.

All of the major companies will buy lunch and provide seminars to develop the staff's knowledge of their products. These ongoing seminars will keep your receptionists and nutritional counselors knowledgeable. Your resort staff also needs to know the importance and significance of low-salt or low-protein diets to their guests' health.

Although all of these programs may not be for every hospital or resort, they should certainly stimulate your thinking. See Appendix 4 for more boarding forms and ideas.

New Technologies & Emerging Trends

7

Computer Monitoring and Other New Toys

As we enter the new millennium, the number of diagnostic toys is increasing. Practice computers are now commonplace; yet just over a decade ago, less than 40 percent of the practices were computerized. The Internet is replacing the fax machine for routine professional communications. State Veterinary Medical Associations are interlined with national veterinary associations by NOAH on the Internet, and the Veterinary Information Network (*www.vin.com*) has over 100 specialists refereeing the special-interest boards on the Internet. Technology is also driving the field of enhanced diagnostics. Just look at what has occurred around us in the recent years of "general" practice:

Dry chemistry systems—easy to use, in-house, blood chemistry screening, including: low-volume systems, electrolyte, thyroid panels, cortisol levels, etc. This has allowed, at a minimum, an increase in preanaesthetic blood screening, sequential laboratory screens, and enhanced emergency medicine diagnostics.

Computer-enhanced endoscopes, opthalmoscopes, otoscopes, surface magnifications, and other fiber optic diagnostic instruments, requiring computer screens in client education areas. This visual education allows enhanced opportunities for clients to see diagnostic changes, such as ear mites moving, retinal vessels, and comparative lesions for growth or reduction.

Audio-stethoscopes—so the consultation room is filled with the beating heart of the patient, and clients can be included in the diagnostic episode. The simple audio sharing of a murmur, or atypical cardiac rhythm, is often the deciding factor in getting approval for appropriate healthcare.

Surface ocular tonometry—hand-held instrumentation for early detection of glaucoma and other eye pressure conditions in horses and companion animals. The slight changes in pressure allow the early diagnostics, so again, the baseline values are critical to successful medical intervention.

Enhanced imaging with not only barium bullets, but with MRI and CT scan capabilities within our own metroplex area. Contrast radiography is underutilized in many practices, often because they are still using hand-tank developing, but the use of advanced imaging is making clients more aware of the alternatives available.

Nutritional advances—we have seen practices start to handle prescription diets as therapy, assigning the nursing staff to follow cases and bring them back into the practice for rechecks at two- to four-week intervals. In 1998, we even saw cartilage therapy diets, cancer diets, and diabetic diets enter the marketplace, as well as holistic pet food, targeted supplements, hedgehog food, and improved avian diets.

Volumetric IV infusion pumps—many of us were trained to "count the drops" and extrapolate, but now we control the flow. Although this is good medicine in all cases and ensures appropriate hydration and therapy, in many small-sized patients, this pump is a critical necessity for efficacious healthcare.

Pulse oximeters, capnometers, and blood pressure monitors are now a screening and monitoring tool, and we even have standards for most species. Many practices include specific levels of monitoring, depending on risk assessment of cases, and others allow the clients to upgrade monitoring levels for an additional fee. The latter will cut our throat in the long run, because it makes monitoring an option rather than a required level of care.

Behavior management—behavior problems are most often the cause of adolescent euthanasia (over 5 million animals a year), with approximately 90 percent of dog owners stating they would like behavior assistance from their veterinarian. A simple awareness (AAHA brochures), the use of a quality head collar (Gentle Leader/Promise®), and staff who are provided the time and healthcare authority to follow this caseload can make a significant difference in client bonding and practice return rates.

Contact cardiac monitors—hand-held, Lead II, rhythm strip monitors, with two, three, or four chest wall contacts (no clips). The utilization of this diagnostic screening instrument will catch early cardiac variances, but more importantly, will be an opportunity for the vet-

FIGURE 7.1

SURGICAL RISK ASSESSMENT

The AAHA Anesthetic/Surgery Log has five levels of risk assessment, and often this column is not used. The five categories are defined as:

1. **Minimal**—healthy patient and client accepted all needed care and wellness protection identified by the veterinary provider

2. **Slight**—healthy patient but client waived or deferred some part of the needed care or wellness protection plan

3. **Moderate**—patient shows some dehydration, medical abnormality, or other form of physical stress

4. **High**—patient shows severe stress, major medical abnormality, which interferes with vital signs or other guarded prognosis condition

5. **Grave**—this patient has a very poor prognosis, and veterinary intervention does not guarantee resolution

erinary provider to again document the needed baseline while establishing the client's acceptance for "age dependent" increases in diagnostic testing intensity.

Pet fat farms—an extension of the respite care programs (respite care, from hospice, for patients with severe medical conditions, where home care providers need a break from the demand). Animals that are overweight are admitted for a two-week, inpatient, refeeding program, with biweekly laboratory screening and home reports. A thinner animal is returned to the client with an appropriate diet already established in the animal's mind.

Senior clubs (elderly clients, not animals)—the need for socialization by seniors is a true opportunity to practice bonding, again operated by the staff and centered on concerned patient care. This basically allows the seniors an evening out at their local veterinary practice once a month.

Stimulation therapy—once thought to be only in the realm of holistic or Oriental therapy, we are seeing a Functional Electrical Stimulation (FES) mobile, hand-held, proven efficacious device used more frequently as a therapy for muscle or tendon injuries in horses.

Oxygen therapy—hyperbaric pressure chambers are appearing, as is recurring oxygen therapy via plastic wrap–enclosed Elizabethan collar for trauma cases, orthopedic wound healing, and neurological patients.

Enhanced surgical equipment, including electro-surgical and laser surgery equipment has been coming down in price and up in quality and ease of utilization. This has added to the microdissection capabilities as well as to flexibility in microsurgical replacement procedures.

Proliferation of private practice specialists within our metroplex communities, no longer university based, so they are tuned into the referring veterinarian. Concurrently, there are more remote service specialists emerging, providing increased diagnostic capabilities within the practice. Not only are they protective of the trust being transferred, but these specialists are not going to do other healthcare, because their clients are the referring practice and the referring veterinarian, and the animal owner is a one-time service.

Ultrasound systems—portable machines that have come down in size and price, lending to screening echocardiology. General practice echocardiology will become commonplace in the new millennium. Although some general practitioners attempt to gain total ultrasound expertise, with different levels of diagnostic success, there are traveling specialists, who come into the practice, as well as central facilities that offer diagnostics from highly trained veterinary providers.

Phosphor plates (receiving the x-rays) are replacing standard x-ray cassettes and film (e.g., Siemens), allowing the computer to dial in the appropriate technique while eliminating processor costs, as well as eliminating all the heavy metal toxicity from x-ray developing. This emerging computerized system has decreased in price tenfold during the 1990s, and if this continues, it will be a viable alternative in specialty practices early in the new millennium.

Recombinant technology—this was saved for last in this list because it redesigns what we have always accepted as vaccination therapy. Scientists have been able to determine the genetic sequences of specific genes by using enzymes of bacterial origin to segment the genetic material of yeast, bacteria, and viruses. This potentially allows mediation of the effects of those segments, and eventually will lead into genetic predisposition and possibly phenotypic modifications. However, right now it already offers three different groups (USDA classifications) for developmental products:

- Type I recombinant (subunit) vaccines—derived from recombinant organisms into which a foreign gene from a specific pathogen has been inserted, then it is propagated and the product of the gene is harvested, purified, and administered as a vaccine (e.g., Lyme disease vaccine). This is currently in the final stages of testing to be used for the new Lyme disease vaccine for humans.
- Type II recombinant (gene-deleted) vaccines—organisms are attenuated through growth under suboptimal conditions (temperature, multiple passages, artificial media, restricted hosts, etc.), causing some genes to be altered and no longer expressed. Specific genes, like those for virulence or pathogenicity, can be deleted from a pathogenic organism, causing the disease. These gene-deleted organisms are less likely to cause the disease, although they still retain the ability to stimulate protective immunity (e.g., pseudo-rabies vaccine).
- Type III recombinant (vectored) vaccines—these consist of nonpathogenic or gene-deleted organisms into which specific genetic material from a pathogen is inserted for the distinct purpose of stimulating a protective immune response when administered to the vaccinate. This recombination takes place in vitro during cocultivation of the vector and a plasmid containing the gene to be inserted (e.g., Newcastle disease, canine distemper, and rabies). Fowl pox viral vectors have proven more efficacious than killed vaccines, are highly specific, and induce a long-lasting immune response.

Most all these new technologies lend themselves to very substantial annual life cycle consultation values in the client's eyes. We really do not care what you call this annual wellness screening in your practice; it is a belief system, not a gimmick. This concept has been discussed elsewhere in this text, in Catanzaro's three-volume series, *Building the Successful Veterinary Practice,* and in the current literature, but the healthcare bottom line is simple. We must return to an annual diagnostic episode so we may prioritize the healthcare plan for our patient. As discussed earlier, this is not an effort to boost the ACT; it is quality healthcare that is tailored to the patient needs (and yes, better medicine is better net income, but that is an outcome of beliefs, not an input of effort). Most of us accept that a patient entering its senior years deserves more diagnostic screening than a young healthy adult, but even young healthy adults need to have some level of diagnostic baseline established in the case of future illness. This is the concept of the annual life cycle consultation—better diagnostics and prioritizing care for subsequent visits, taking smaller bites of the client's discretionary income while ensuring the patient is offered the care that is needed for their current needs. This even applies to traveling pets (weekends, vacations, etc.) as well as those that have increased potential contacts (parks, dog or cat shows, nose-to-nose fence time, etc.). If you do not ask, you will never know!

Gatekeeper Referrals

So the emerging equipment technologies can be used in a general practice, but what of the emerging service technologies? Besides the ideas offered in *Building the Successful Veterinary Practice: Innovation & Creativity* (Volume 3), consider the general practice affiliations we are already seeing:

Buying co-ops—the veterinarians in the Canadian provinces have taken this to an art form, with dividends and interactive boards. In specific communities like Las Vegas and the Twin Cities, we have seen some local practice leaders network very effectively for the best buy when they combine their purchases. We are beginning to see logic and reason entering the regional and national buying co-ops in the United States. As this trend continues, participation will increase, as will the savings.

Shared equipment—in some communities, usually middle-sized communities with less than a dozen practices, sharing scarce diagnostic resources is becoming more common. One practice has an endoscope, another has a 500 mA x-ray machine, another has a blood chemistry system, and another has a computerized cardiac screening system; they use a shared ambulance service to move patients behind the scenes, so the site of shared healthcare diagnostic services is transparent to the clients.

Networked staff sharing—again, this is a limited experience at present, usually seen with practices within the same common interest environment, whether it be an emergency practice, shared associate doctor, or similar shared human resource situation.

Emergency practices—often a share-based cooperative, but sometimes just a users group, with a common outcome goal (e.g., freedom from night call). The challenge in many communities, it requires about 26 full-time equivalent (FTE) veterinarians to support a stand-alone emergency practice, and this density is not available to refer clients, so a rotary is needed. To establish a rotary, trust is required between colleagues, and in some cases, the lack of trust prevents sharing, reducing the economies of scale that increase net.

New owner orientation, pet kindergarten, puppy clubs, kitten carrier classes and similar awareness and socialization programs are usually started before the client is aware of behavior management needs. Many practices are offering new owner orientation through adoption centers and pet stores, providing a short, staff-operated, one-hour, courtesy weekend program, within two weeks of a dated seller-completed certificate, as a pet protection effort (and just coincidentally, starts early client bonding).

Boarding facilities—no longer just runs in the country, they are affiliating with veterinary practices and have gone beyond long rows of cage banks. They now include veterinary supervised boarding (e.g., hospice respite care), cat condos, exploration zones, pet partners instead of attendants, VIP suites with television and brass beds, play time, and sometimes, provided with optional people time, swim time, and even specially blended, animal friendly, afternoon yogurt treats.

Grooming facilities—once a garage or basement operation, or maybe a table in the back of a veterinary clinic with someone with clippers and scissors doing summer cuts, more trained groomers are affiliating with veterinary practices. We are seeing a beauty salon atmosphere, with ribbons, fragrances, decorated booths, underlit tables, and custom grooming cuts, all with specialized callbacks and frequent grooming programs that offer a per cut bargain when the client stays on schedule.

Pet boutiques—the resale shelves have given way to upscale retail activities, with custom jewelry and curios, as well as the latest in pet attire and accessories ... and yes, custom and prescription foods are still available.

Special interest practices in eyes, dentistry, cardiology, orthopedics, etc., have started to emerge in communities with a dozen or so practices. This is usually too small for a specialty practice but large enough for the senior players to have mutual respect and the time to develop special interests, so trusted referrals are possible for everyone.

Exotic patient referrals—the atypical, alternative pet requires special equipment, a special holding facility, and most often, special continuing education to stay current with the trends (e.g., misting systems for iguanas in the arid west). Most practices are more than happy to refer an expensive parrot, the pot-bellied pig, a poisonous reptile, pygmy goats, or fish to someone who likes those kinds of critters.

Allergy interests—the development of referral allergy services (like V.A.R.L.), which provide courtesy consultations as a matter of client service, has increased the use of animal specific allergy medications that become life of patient refills (increase in traffic and net, for virtually no cost, after the initial diagnostic episode).

The Use of Specialists to Build Your Practice

The more diagnostics you can do in-house, the better medicine and surgery you can practice, but there are various ways to utilize the specialist services emerging in this profession. The 1970s saw our university-based teaching hospitals turning out practitioners, but then class sizes increased (response to the tax dollar demands) and the "me generation" drove a self-centered emphasis in veterinary healthcare excellence. Student-based National Veterinary Association linkages in the university teaching hospital gave way to specialty groups in the veterinary teaching hospitals in the 1980s. Specialization became the mark of the academic world by the 1990s. New graduates proliferated, as did practices around the teaching hospitals. Primary care caseload gave way to tertiary care caseload, feeding the specialist needs in the university veterinary teaching hospital settings. New graduates were skilled in tertiary care, but many had not seen a cat abscess, broken nail, grass awn, or even done a basic dental hygiene cleaning. Thanks to the academic system, residents and interns have been graduating faster than the teaching hospitals can absorb them. There are now specialty practices emerging in most metroplex areas, and some of the specialists are even looking outside the standard metroplex for a quality-of-life location to practice.

Specialization infers a board certification, but in fact, often involves board-qualified veterinarians. This leads to the general practice having a special interest in certain types of procedures or certain species. This trend will increase in the next millennium, not decrease, so what is perceived today as emerging may be commonplace tomorrow.

The first special-interest practice is almost becoming a traditional method—refer to an emergency practice during the hours you do not want to be on call to your clients. Some practices in limited density areas are addressing this demand by becoming twenty-four hour practices, often with a technician serving a screening role during the dark-of-night hours. Another option to this weekend and evening special-interest practice scope, usually in smaller communities, is to develop a rotary, where a few practices agree to cooperate and see each other's out-of-hours cases on an equitable rotation schedule. This requires ethical behavior on each participant's part (they do not steal clients and do not offer routine wellness care during the emergency episode), as well as a trust in the level of veterinary healthcare being offered by the other participating veterinary practices.

Another emerging special-interest practice is the atypical pet, what we call exotics. Iguanas, birds, fish, even spiders and snakes—all can become alternative pets. Some practices have installed an "exotic closet"; a small space with controlled humidity and temperature, while others have procured many retiring incubators from local human hospitals. In both cases, the husbandry awareness is making the difference when trying to differentiate the practice in the eyes of the potential clients.

As discussed earlier, in moderate sized communities with less than 20 veterinarians in practices, there is often the old style colleague trust, which allows practices to share resources in equipment, special interests, and rotary emergency call services. Sometimes this occurs in larger communities, such as Buffalo or Seattle, but that has been the exception rather than the rule. We hope the future sees our profession returning to the status of colleagues rather than competitors. That will be a pivotal role provided by the local veterinary associations (the ones that want to survive in the new millennium).

The traveling specialist has expanded this past decade, sometimes to multiple states away. They are contracted to come into a practice and perform their specialty for a few days to a week. Some states, like Nevada, have even waived state licensure requirements for these traveling specialists, as long as they restrict their services to their board-certified specialty. If your state or province allows this form of specialist referral, now is the time to network with specialists in other communities or states and develop a referral system of sponsorship so clients are brought back into your own facility to see the traveling specialist. In a community of colleagues, this allows each practice to develop a sponsorship linkage with a specific specialty and increase the cross-referrals between practices, thereby raising the quality bar concurrent with the income levels derived with sponsorship of specialized care providers.

So with these trends placed on the table, what is next? Is there a future for veterinarians postresidency? If the schools continue to allow the old mentality of "You can't afford to do this in practice," the future is dim. Some schools, like Tufts, have been evolving their way into partnerships with private practice, placing interns and residents into a for-profit environment for some or all of their advanced training. This effort is to be applauded. I was standing in one practice when the head of the Tufts program came in and saw the resident who had been working in a private, for-profit, emergency practice for six months. He asked, "How are you doing?" The reply was rapid, and targeted, "I have less than $2,000 accounts receivable after six months!" As the silence enveloped the exchange, I interceded with accolades, which were quickly followed by similar appreciation by the Tufts professors as well as the practice owners. A resident who understood the economics of emergency practice—amazing! This is the eye-opening experience our young residents really need, because it allows them to better understand private practice and for-profit veterinary healthcare delivery operations.

Have you contacted your university teaching hospital with the availability of externships, preceptorships, internships, or even residency opportunities if there is a board-certified specialist or two on staff? This is a great method to prescreen team members for the future! In some communities, this linkage is provided to the local high school or junior college in business relations and marketing, as well as in veterinary medicine disciplines. In one community, we even interlinked with a local vo-tech nursing school (human) for work-study opportunities for their students, and many became technician assistants instead of entering human healthcare.

Other Emerging Trends

The outpatient nurse appointment is talked about so often that many times we forget that it is an evolving activity. The position of outpatient nurse is based on someone who can walk, chew gum, and communicate effectively with clients—all at the same time. They do not need a large bag of skills; rather, they need a *very* large bag of options based on the knowledge of the practice. They need to have an attitude of caring, compassion, and can-do. And while we are at it, we call them *nurses* because that is a term our clients automatically associate with doctors, while a *technician* infers that they work with a "small animal repair person." Why do clients want to see the doctor? We have never given them other expectations. The practices that produce in excess of $500,000 per doctor use a nursing staff as veterinary extenders. The ones that stay below $300,000 per doctor usually do not develop the staff; the doctors try to do it all themselves. Consider these as just a few options to consider when developing the healthcare team in your practice:

- Outpatient nurses
- Inpatient nurses
- Nutritional advisors
- Dental hygiene specialists
- Parasite prevention & control counselors
- Behavior management aides
- Wellness nurses
- Vaccination clinic providers
- ICU/CCU nurses
- Client outreach agents
- Surgical nurses
- Nurse anesthetists
- Birthing coaches

In some metroplex communities a few companion animal veterinary practices are evolving into gatekeepers of the specialty practices in the area. They deal in wellness and diagnostics and refer almost every inpatient or challenging case to a specialist. This may sound unusual, until you think of the litigation emerging on the two coasts concerning the failure to offer the client a referral to a specialist. We have even seen clients enter emergency practices and request a board-certified surgeon for a trauma case. This is an emerging trend, and will likely never be common in rural communities. In metroplex communities, be aware of the trend!

Distance learning is increasing, not only for doctors but also for staff. There are certified veterinary technician programs being offered on-line; Veterinary Information Network (VIN) or NOAH usually has a listing of the AVMA-certified technician programs. This means the staff member can work full time in your practice, attend classes on the computer at their own pace, and earn a degree that permits them to apply to take state boards. If technical assistants are provided this level of continuing education, turnover decreases, pride in performance increases, and interactive healthcare delivery discussions increase.

Computer-assisted instruction for clients has been increasing within the practices, as has the use of the Internet by clients. There are many programs, the newest being interactive CD-ROM systems, becoming available for client education; these are usually stand alone, but clients should never be allowed to "stand alone" during the information-sharing experience. Real people who care about the patient and client are needed to explain any automated presentation. It is not uncommon for clients to bring a set of Internet articles about a specific problem into the practice and expect the veterinary provider to be fully aware of the current opinions on the Internet. This is both good and bad, depending on how the practice monitors the Internet and handles the client's questions. A full disclosure of specialist options often shortcuts the client, because they become aware of the levels of care available.

The sabbatical is increasing in multiowner private practices, and this trend is exciting. One partner is allowed to leave for an extended period of time, usually months at a time, on a rotational basis. The level of income may not be decreased, but often the departing doctor hires his own professional replacement from the established cash flow of the sabbatical package. Regardless, the secret here is that the sabbatical must keep the doctor out of the practice for the required amount of time. In some cases, much of this time is spent on refresher courses with specialists, a university veterinary teaching hospital, or even a local community hospital. In other cases, the time is spent with family traveling, with a hobby, or in other unwind activities of the doctor's choosing. It is easy to see that a mix and match of activities, professional and personal, makes the sabbatical a great break from the grind of practice ownership.

The practice business team is actually a new concept and has been ignored when developing most veterinary practices. In most successful small businesses, a team of experts advises the owner; veterinary practice owners are no different. The commercial banker advises the business on loans, lines of credit, and community trends. Participation in local civic clubs (Rotary, Kiwanis, Optimists, Lions, etc.) makes the community-wide contacts needed for effective business resources. The tax accountant is essential and should be well versed in professional practices and the tax code affecting them; they only advise the internal bookkeeper on an as needed basis. The practice attorney should not be a generalist, but rather a professional corporation attorney who can advise on structure, buy-sell, contracts, and related legal issues. The veterinary-exclusive practice consultant should match the practice personality, be operationally in tune with the trends of the practice and community and be ready to advise the attorney, banker, and accountant on issues of practice importance. This team of consultants should become the often-used resources for program-based decisions, capital expense procurement advice, and human resource organizational behavior assistance. Quarterly review of operational data by each of these business team members may not be required, but quarterly review by at least one of the business team resources should be considered a requirement of operation. All should be involved with a practice review annually, usually in conjunction with the annual planning retreat (see Chapter 4 of *Building the Successful Veterinary Practice: Programs & Procedures*, Volume 2).

Strategic Assessment—Putting It All Together

Please do not try! Emerging trends are just that, emerging. They are not for everyone. They will not fit all communities. They cannot be made to work when the environment (internal or external) will not support the program. What is needed is a targeted strategic assessment each year.

What is a strategic assessment for a veterinary practice? It is an assessment of the external opportunities as well as the external threats. The threats and opportunities cannot be manipulated by the practice. However, they can be observed and categorized, and they can be used to adjust internal activities. Internally, a practice has strengths and weaknesses that must be strategically assessed. The facility, the location, the access, the staff skills, the scope of services, equipment resources, knowledge levels, and core values and belief systems, are all internal. Weakness or strength is often a factor of positive mental attitude.

One of the tools that has proven most useful to those who like to do strategic assessments is building the four quadrant box. Each quadrant represents one factor of the strategic assessment—opportunity, threat, strength, or weakness. Each box represents *only* one issue, one challenge, or one concern. The four elements are brainstormed by the team for each of the four assessment elements in a free thought and association process. In this process, there are no vetoes and no bias is allowed; extra assessment blocks (four quadrant sheets) may be required if the programs, concerns, or challenges are reidentified as multielement issues. It does not matter which quadrant is opportunity, threat, strength, or weakness, as long as you draw the box and identify the quadrants the same each time. Some elements may require double entries, such as a "well-oiled, harmonious, practice team." This team may have been built under the old model where only doctors did outpatient nursing. The internal harmony strength becomes a weakness when addressing the outpatient nurse duties. The new homes being built within the catchment area may be an external opportunity for new clients, but the facility capabilities may already be maximized, making the increased demand an internal weakness. Do not be structured; write it all down. After the quadrants are filled and the opinions are categorized, then discuss what the practice should do in the future. Forward thinking, no excuses, and never blaming, is the key to strategic assessment activities!

The wonderful thing about this chapter is that much of it will be out of date before the book is published. Today's innovation is tomorrow's mediocrity. Metaphane gave way to halothane, which gave way to isoflurane, and anesthetic protocols continue to change every day. We all have used pain medication, but pain scoring is an emerging requirement of quality healthcare. Everyone knows food is required for survival, but only the most comprehensive practices handle it as a medical necessity, which includes sequential weights, annual blood chemistries, and nutritional scoring for inpatients. The cutting edge requires constant honing. The proactive practice does not change because others have; it changes because the community and clients have shown a need. The veterinary practice of the new millennium is no longer just reactive to stress; it causes chaos in the professional community by being a leader in innovation and creativity. So, empower the practice team members, assess the emerging community needs, and start the innovation engine for the new millennium. Enjoy the ride; it will be exciting!

APPENDIX 1

Programs

PROGRAMS WORK SHEET

Program for: PUPPY

ITEM	REG. CHG.	VISIT 1 6-8 weeks	VISIT 2 9-12 weeks	VISIT 3 13-15 weeks	VISIT 4 6-18 weeks
PE/Consult		•		•	
DHPPC		•	•	•	•
Bordetella		•			
Lyme				•	•
Rabies					•
Fecal		•			•
Deworm		•	•	•	•
Rx sentinel		•			
Weight		•	•	•	•
Behavioral consult		•			•
Set up neuter					•
DISCOUNT					
FREE GOODS					
COST TO CLIENT					

PROGRAMS WORK SHEET

Program for: KITTEN

ITEM	REG. CHG.	VISIT 1 6-8 weeks	VISIT 2 9-12 weeks	VISIT 3 13-15 weeks	VISIT 4 6-18 weeks
PE/Consult		•		•	
FVRCP		•	•	•	
FeLV			•	•	
FIP					• +4 wk
Rabies				•	•
FeLV test		•			
Fecal		•			•
Deworm		•	•	•	•
Rx program		•			
Weight		•	•	•	•
Set up neuter					•
DISCOUNT					
FREE GOODS					
COST TO CLIENT					

PROGRAMS WORK SHEET

Program for: YOUNG ADULT (1–5 YEARS), DOG OR CAT

ITEM	REG. CHG.	LEVEL 1	LEVEL 2	LEVEL 3	OPTIONS
PE/Consult		•	•	•	•
FVRCP DHPPC		•	•	•	•
FeLV Bordetella		•	•	•	•
FIP Lyme		•	•	•	•
Rabies		• If needed	• If needed	• If needed	• If needed
FeLV/FIV test Heartworm test		•	•	•	•
Fecal		•	•	•	•
Deworm		•	•	•	•
Rx program Rx sentinel		•	•	•	•
Weight		•	•	•	•
Screening blood test		4 tests	6 tests	12 tests	Thyroid
Urinalysis			•	•	
Ld. II EKG					•
Hip rads					•
Tear test			•	•	
Glaucoma (IOP) screen			•	•	
Dental disease screen		•	•	•	
DISCOUNT			10%	15%	
FREE GOODS					
COST TO CLIENT					

PROGRAMS WORK SHEET

Program for: MIDDLE AGE (6–8 YEARS), DOG OR CAT

ITEM	REG. CHG.	LEVEL 1	LEVEL 2	LEVEL 3	OPTIONS
PE/Consult		•	•	•	
FVRCP DHPPC		•	•	•	
FeLV Bordetella		•	•	•	
FIP Lyme		•	•	•	
Rabies		• If needed	• If needed	• If needed	
FeLV/FIV test Heartworm test		•	•	•	
Fecal		•	•	•	
Deworm		•	•	•	
Rx program Rx sentinel		•	•	•	
Weight		•	•	•	
Screening blood test		6 tests	12 tests	Thyroid	
Urinalysis		•	•	•	
Ld. II EKG		•	•	•	
Hip rads					•
Tear test			•	•	
Glaucoma (IOP) screen			•	•	
Dental disease screen		•	•	•	
DISCOUNT			10%	15%	
FREE GOODS					
COST TO CLIENT					

PROGRAMS WORK SHEET

Program for: OLDER ADULT (>9 YEARS), DOG OR CAT

ITEM	REG. CHG.	LEVEL 1	LEVEL 2	LEVEL 3	OPTIONS
PE/Consult		•	•	•	
FVRCP DHPPC		•	•	•	
FeLV Bordetella		•	•	•	
FIP Lyme		•	•	•	
Rabies		• If needed	• If needed	• If needed	
FeLV/FIV test Heartworm test		•	•	•	
Fecal		•	•	•	
Deworm		•	•	•	
Rx program Rx sentinel		•	•	•	
Weight		•	•	•	
Screening blood test		12 tests	Thyroid	12 tests Thyroid	
Urinalysis		•	•	•	
Ld. II EKG		•	•	6 lead	
Hip/back rads					•
Chest rads				•	
Tear test		•	•	•	
Glaucoma (IOP) screen		•	•	•	
Dental disease screen		•	•	•	
DISCOUNT					
FREE GOODS					
COST TO CLIENT					

Program for: SKIN DISEASES

ITEM	REG. CHG.	LEVEL 1	LEVEL 2	LEVEL 3	LEVEL 4
PE/Consult		•	•	•	•
Skin scrape		•	•	•	•
Skin cytology			•	•	•
Fungal culture		•	•	•	•
Injection		•	•	•	•
Injection			• (e.g., Ivermectin)	•	•
Oral Rx		•	•	•	•
Oral Rx		•	•	•	•
Topical			•	•	•
Shampoo		•	•	•	•
Flea control— oral/injectable		•	10% off	10 % off	15% off
Flea control— topical		•	10% off	10 % off	15% off
Diet supplement			•	•	•
Sedate				•	•
Biopsy				•	•
Skin C & S				•	•
Allergy test					•
Antigens					•
Blood profile				•	•
Thryoid profile					•
Adrenal profile					option
Rechecks		2 free	4 free	6 free	8 free
DISCOUNT					
FREE GOODS					
COST TO CLIENT					

PROGRAMS WORK SHEET

Program for: EAR DISEASES

ITEM	REG. CHG.	LEVEL 1	LEVEL 2	LEVEL 3	LEVEL 4
PE/Consult		•	•	•	•
Skin scrape			•	•	•
Ear cytology		•	•	•	•
Fungal culture			•	•	•
Injection		•	•	•	•
Injection			• (e.g., Ivermectin)	•	•
Oral Rx		•	•	•	•
Oral Rx			•	•	•
Topical		•	•	•	•
Topical			•	•	•
Ear cleaning		•	•	•	•
Flea control—oral/injectable			10% off	10 % off	15% off
Flea control—topical			10% off	10 % off	15% off
Diet supplement			•	•	•
Sedate				•	•
Ear flush				•	•
Ear C & S				•	•
Allergy test					•
Antigens					•
Blood profile				•	•
Thryoid profile					•
Adrenal profile					option

Program for: EAR DISEASES *(continued)*

ITEM	REG. CHG.	LEVEL 1	LEVEL 2	LEVEL 3	LEVEL 4
Rechecks		2 free	4 free	6 free	8 free
Repeat ear cytology		2 free	4 free	6 free	8 free
Rx refills		10% off	12 % off	15% off	15% off
Sedate and flush			Inc. 2	Inc. 3	Inc. 4
Lateral ear Sx					$200 off
DISCOUNT					
FREE GOODS					
COST TO CLIENT					

PROGRAMS WORK SHEET

Program for: CHRONIC RENAL FAILURE

ITEM	REG. CHG.	LEVEL 1	LEVEL 2	LEVEL 3	LEVEL 4
PE/Consult		•	•	•	•
Laboratory		•	•	•	•
Urinalysis		•	•	•	•
Radiographs			•	•	•
Urine MIC			•	•	•
IV catheter				•	•
Hospitalization				•	•
Fluids				•	•
Injections				•	•
Diet		•	•	•	•
Rechecks		**1 free**	**3 free**	**4 free**	**6 free**
Recheck lab		1 included (PCV, Bun, Creat, Phos only)	2 included (PCV, Bun Creat Phos only)	4 included **Mini Profiles**	4 included **Full Profiles**
SQ fluids at home		•	**4 liters**	**8 liters**	**12 liters**
Euthanasia					**N/C**
DISCOUNT					
FREE GOODS					
COST TO CLIENT					

PROGRAMS WORK SHEET

Program for: HEART MURMUR/CHF

ITEM	REG. CHG.	LEVEL 1	LEVEL 2	LEVEL 3	LEVEL 4
PE/Consult		•	•	•	•
Chest rads		•	•	•	•
EKG		•	•	•	•
Lab profile		•	•	•	•
Urinalysis		•	•	•	•
Ultrasound			•	•	•
Oral Rx		•	•	•	•
Oral Rx			•	•	•
Diet			•	•	•
Rechecks		Inc. 1	Inc. 2	Inc. 4	Inc. 6
Recheck lab			Inc. 1	Inc. 2	Inc. 3
Recheck rads			Inc. 1 ×	Inc. 2 ×	Inc. 3 ×
Recheck EKG			Inc. 1 ×	Inc. 2 ×	Inc. 3 ×
Recheck U.S.					Inc. 1 ×
DISCOUNT					
FREE GOODS					
COST TO CLIENT					

PROGRAMS WORK SHEET

Program for: GLAUCOMA

ITEM	REG. CHG.	LEVEL 1	LEVEL 2	LEVEL 3	LEVEL 4
PE/Consult		•	•	•	•
STT		•	•	•	•
IOP		•	•	•	•
Florestain		•	•	•	•
Lab profile			6 test	Full	Thyroid
U/A			•	•	•
Oral Rx		•	•	•	•
Oral Rx			•	•	•
Topical Rx		•	•	•	•
Topical Rx			•	•	•
Recheck		1×	2×	4×	6×
Recheck IOP		1×	2×	4×	6×
Rx refill		1×	2×	4×	6×
Enucleation Sx					$100 off
DISCOUNT					
FREE GOODS					
COST TO CLIENT					

PROGRAMS WORK SHEET

Program for: K C S

ITEM	REG. CHG.	LEVEL 1	LEVEL 2	LEVEL 3	LEVEL 4
PE/Consult		•	•	•	•
STT		•	•	•	•
IOP		•	•	•	•
Florestain		•	•	•	•
Lab profile			6 test	Full	Thyroid
U/A			•	•	•
Oral Rx		•	•	•	•
Oral Rx		•	•	•	•
Topical Rx		•	•	•	•
Topical Rx		•	•	•	•
Recheck		1×	2×	4×	6×
Recheck STT		1×	2×	4×	6×
Rx refills		1×	2×	4×	6×
DISCOUNT					
FREE GOODS					
COST TO CLIENT					

PROGRAMS WORK SHEET

Program for: CORNEAL ULCERS

ITEM	REG. CHG.	LEVEL 1	LEVEL 2	LEVEL 3	LEVEL 4
PE/Consult		•	•	•	•
IOP		•	•	•	•
STT			•	•	•
Florestain		•	•	•	•
Lab profile				•	•
U/A				•	•
Topical Rx		•	•	•	•
Topical Rx			•	•	•
Oral Rx			•	•	•
Oral Rx				•	•
Rechecks		Inc. 1	Inc. 2	Inc. 3	Inc. 4
Recheck Florestain		Inc. 1	Inc. 2	Inc. 3	Inc. 4
Topical anesth.				•	•
Corneal debridement				•	•
Sedate				•	•
Third eyelid flap					•
DISCOUNT					
FREE GOODS					
COST TO CLIENT					

Program for: CHEMOTHERAPY

ITEM	REG. CHG.	LEVEL 1	LEVEL 2	LEVEL 3	LEVEL 4
PE/Consult		•	•	•	•
Lab profile		•	•	•	•
U/A		•	•	•	•
Rads		•	•	•	•
IV catheter			•	•	•
Fluids			•	•	•
Injectable			•	•	•
Injectable				•	•
Oral Rx			•	•	•
Oral Rx				•	•
Rechecks			1×	2×	4×
Recheck lab			1×	2×	4×
Recheck rads				1×	2×
Rx refills			10%	12%	15%
DISCOUNT					
FREE GOODS					
COST TO CLIENT					

DENTAL PROGRAMS

The following services are anticipated and included in the outlined levels of care. This chart is for the purpose of generating estimates only. Actual services will be determined and provided as deemed appropriate by the veterinarian at the time of anesthesia and thorough exam. The estimate given will be honored for routine care. If extraordinary conditions are found upon anesthesia and full exam, the client will be consulted before additional work proceeds and additional costs are incurred.

	FEE	LEVEL 1	LEVEL 2	LEVEL 3	LEVEL 4
Preanesthetic lab work	Varies	•	•	•	•
Preanesthetic exam		•	•	•	•
Induction		•	•	•	•
Isoflurane anesthesia		•	•	•	•
Chart teeth		•	•	•	•
Clean		•	•	•	•
Polish		•	•	•	•
Fluoride		•	•	•	•
Postanesthesia monitor			•	•	•
Antibiotic injection				•	•
Anti-pain injection				•	•
Oral antibiotics TGH					•
Oral pain meds TGH					+/-
Radiographs					+/-
Single root extractions					+/-
Carnasal extraction $4.25/m	8–12 min.				
Canine extraction $4.25/m	10–20 min.				
Home care instruction kit		•	•	•	•
Dental care samples		•	•	•	•
Coupon for brush training		•	•	•	•
Disc dental products 6 mo.		•	•	•	•

Note that the time required for cleaning the teeth increases with each level of dental care. This time factor is a major contributor to the costs of the procedures in addition to the points outlined above.

BEHAVIOR MANAGEMENT PROGRAMS

"Practice success in the new millennium lies in a veterinary healthcare team embracing patient advocacy and client-centered service, telling animal stewards what is needed (❑) for wellness, and then being quiet and listening to the client about what they want to access today."

—Thomas E. Catanzaro, DVM, MHA, FACHE

Accountable Team Member: _____ Start Date: _____

PET NEEDS   (Index)

❑ **FIRST VISIT (Kitten/Puppy)**
  ❑ House training (poster)
  ❑ Litter box program
  ❑ Odor control/stain removal
  ❑ Husbandry
  ❑

❑ **SECOND VISIT (socialization)**
  ❑ Head collar   (Campbell)
  ❑ Scat mat
  ❑ Slap trap
  ❑ Kong toy
  ❑

❑ **Traveling with Your Pet (handout)**
  ❑ Sedation
  ❑ Kennels
  ❑

❑ **Separation Anxiety**
  ❑ Clomicalm
  ❑ Kong toy
  ❑ Behavior consultant   (AVMA)
  ❑

❑ **Behavior Challenges**
  ❑ Staff consultation ($15–$20)
  ❑ AAHA booklets   (AAHA)
  ❑ Behavior consultant   (AVMA)
  ❑

APPENDIX 2

Protocols and Bundles

Abscess—Major
Office Call
Isoflurane (First 20 min)
Isoflurane (Additional 20 min)
Drain Tube(s)
IV Catheter & Insertion
Administration Set
Lactated Ringer's Solution
Amoxi—Inject
Amoxicillin 400 mg. tabs
Chlorhexi-Derm Flush 12 oz.
Hospitalization
Suture Incision/Laceration
ECG Monitoring
Standard O.R. Setup
Preanesthetic Screen
Induce Anesthesia
Major Surgical Pack

Abscess—Minor
Office Call
Isoflurane (First 20 min)
Drain Tube(s)
Amoxicillin 15 ml liquid
Chlorhexi-Derm Flush 4 oz.
Amoxi—Inject
ECG Monitoring
Standard O.R. Setup
Preanesthetic Screen
Minor Surgical Pack
Induce Anesthesia
Hospitalization

Amputate Digit
Office Call
Radiograph—1st
Additional Radiograph
Isoflurane (First 20 min)
Isoflurane (Add'l 20 min)
IV Catheter & Insertion
Lactated Ringer's Mix
Administration Set
Hospitalization
Amputation—Digit
Standard O.R. Setup
ECG Monitoring
Preanesthetic Screen
Cephalothin Sodium Inj
Cephalexin 500 mg.
3M C/C Med Collar—Size 30
Induce Anesthesia
Major Surgical Pack

Amputate Front Limb
Office Call
Radiograph—1st
Additional Radiograph
Isoflurane (First 20 min)
Isoflurane (Add'l 20 min)

IV Catheter & Insertion
Lactated Ringer's Solution
Administration Set
Hospitalization
Amputation—Front leg
Cephelexin 500 mg.
Cephalothin Sodium Inj.
Standard O.R. Setup
ECG Monitoring
Preanesthetic Screen
Torbugesic
Induce Anesthesia
Major Surgical Pack
Fentanyl Patch

Amputate Rear Leg
Office Call
Radiograph—1st
Additional Radiograph
Isoflurane (First 20 min)
Isolfurane (Add'l 20 min)
Torbugesic
IV Catheter & Insertion
Lactated Ringer's Solution
Administration Set
Hospitalization
Amputation—Rear Leg
Clindamycin 150 mg.
Amoxi—Inject
Standard O.R. Setup
ECG Monitoring
Preanesthetic Screen
Fentanyl Patch

Anal Gland Removal
Office Call
Isoflurane (First 20 min)
Isoflurane (Add'l 20 min)
IV Catheter & Insertion
Lactated Ringer's Solution
Administration Set
Hospitalization
Anal Sac Removal
Amoxi—Inject
Amoxicillin 400 mg. tabs
3M C/C Med Collar—Size 17
Standard O.R. Setup
ECG Monitoring
Preanesthetic Screen
Induce Anesthesia
Major Surgical Pack
Torbugesic
Fentanyl Patch

Caesarian Section—Canine
Office Call
Standard O.R. Setup
ECG Monitoring
Tube Feeding

Isoflurane (First 20 min)
Isoflurane (Add'l 20 min)
Oxygen Therapy
IV Catheter & Insertion
Lactated Ringer's Mix
Administration Set
Hospitalization
Caesarian Section—Canine
Amoxicillin 400 mg. tabs
Amoxi—Inject
Oxytocin Inj.
Dopram-V Injection
Radiograph—1st
Preanesthetic Screen
Additional Radiograph
Induce Anesthesia
Major Surgical Pack
Resuscitate Puppies

Caesarian Section—Feline
Office Call
Standard O.R. Setup
ECG Monitoring
Tube Feeding
Isoflurane (First 20 min)
Isoflurane (Add'l 20 min)
Oxygen Therapy
IV Catheter & Insertion
Lactated Ringer's Mix
Administration Set
Hospitalization
Caesarian Section—Feline
Amoxicillin 100 mg. tabs
Amoxi—Inject
Oxytocin Inj.
Dopram-V Injection
Radiograph—1st
Preanesthetic Screen
Additional Radiograph
Induce Anesthesia
Major Surgical Pack

Cherry Eye Restoration (single)
Office Call
Standard O.R. Setup
ECG Monitoring
Isoflurane (First 20 min)
Isoflurane (Add'l 20 min)
Restore Third Eyelid
BNPH
Preanesthetic Screen
Prednisone Injection
Minor Surgical Pack
Hospitalization
Induce Anesthesia

Cherry Eye Restored (bilateral)
Office Call
Standard O.R. Setup

ECG Monitoring
Isoflurane (First 20 min)
Isoflurane (Add'l 20 min)
Restore Third Eyelid Bilateral
BNPH
Preanesthetic Screen
Prednisone Injection
Hospitalization
Minor Surgical Pack
Induce Anesthesia

Corneal Laceration
Office Call
Standard O.R. Setup
ECG Monitoring
Stain Eye
Isoflurane (First 20 min)
Isoflurane (Add'l 20 min)
Hospitalization
Eye Surgery
Tarsorrophy & 3rd Eyelid Flap
Baytril 68 mg.
Baytril Injectable
Atropine Ophthalmic Drops
BNP
Preanesthetic Screen
Major Surgical Pack

Corrective Ear Surgery
Office Call
Standard O.R. Setup
ECG Monitoring
Isoflurane (First 20 min)
Isoflurane (Add'l 20 min)
Bandage Ear Crop
Corrective Ear Surgery
Large Kennel
Preanesthetic Screen
Hospitalization
Major Surgical Pack
Amoxi—Inject
Induce Anesthesia

Critical Care
Office Call
Dexamethasone Sodium Phosphate
Hospitalization
Thorax (2 views)
Abdomen (2 views)
Extremity (2 views)
IV Catheter & Insertion
Administration Set
Lactated Ringer's Solution
Amoxi—Inject
Complete Blood Count (CBC)
Oxygen Therapy
Biochemistry Profile
Urinalysis/Sediment Exam
ECG—Routine

Cruciate Reconstruction
Office Call
Standard O.R. Setup
ECG Monitoring
Robert Jones Bandage-Med.
Radiograph—1st
Additional Radiograph
Isoflurane (First 20 min)
Isoflurane (Add'l 20 min)
IV Catheter & Insertion
Lactated Ringer's Solution
Administration Set
Hospitalization
Repair Torn Cruciate Ligament
Amoxicillin 400 mg. tabs
Amoxi—Inject
Preanesthetic Screen
Torbugesic
Major Surgical Pack
Induce Anesthesia
Fentanyl Patch

Cystitis—Canine
Office Call
Urinalysis/Sediment Exam
Radiograph—1st
Additional Radiograph
C/D K-9 10#
Amoxicillin 400 mg. tabs
Amoxi—Inject
Prednisone Injection
Cystocentesis
Complete Blood Count (CBC)
Biochemistry Profile

Cystotomy
Office Call
Standard O.R. Setup
ECG Monitoring
Urinalysis/Sediment Exam
Urinary Calculi Analysis
Radiograph—1st
Additional Radiograph
Isoflurane (First 20 min)
Isoflurane (Add'l 20 min)
IV Catheter & Insertion
Saline Solution (0.9% NaCl)
Administration Set
Hospitalization
Cystotomy
C/D K-9 10#
Amoxicillin 400 mg. tabs
Amoxi—Inject
Prednisone Injection
Indwelling Urinary Catheter
Preanesthetic Screen
Major Surgical Pack
Induce Anesthesia

Torbugesic
Fentanyl Patch

Debark
Office Call
Standard O.R. Setup
ECG Monitoring
Isoflurane (First 20 min)
Isoflurane (Add'l 20 min)
Debark—Oral
Amoxicillin 400 mg. tabs
Amoxi—Inject
Prednisone 20 mg. tabs
Prednisone Injection
Preanesthetic Screen
Acepromazine 25 mg.
Hospitalization
Major Surgical Pack
Induce Anesthesia

Dental—Feline
Office Call—Courtesy
Induce Anesthesia
Isoflurane (First 20 min)
Isoflurane (Add'l 20 min)
Feline Scale & Polish
Fluoride Treatment
ECG Monitoring
Preanesthetic Screen
Clindamycin Inj.
Clindamycin Aquadrops 20 ml
Maxiguard—Feline

Dental—Severe
Office Call—Courtesy
Induce Anesthesia
Isoflurane (First 20 min)
Isoflurane (Add'l 20 min)
Clindamycin Inj.
Fluoride Treatment
Canine Scale & Polish—Severe
ECG Monitoring
Preanesthetic Screen
IV Catheter & Insertion
Lactated Ringer's Solution
Clindamycin 75 mg.
Maxiguard Gel 4 oz.
Multiple Extractions

Dewclaws—Adult
Office Call
Standard O.R. Setup
ECG Monitoring
Bandage—Small
Isoflurane (First 20 min)
Remove Dewclaws
Amoxicillin 400 mg. tabs
Amoxi—Inject
Preanesthetic Screen
Isoflurane (Add'l 20 min)

Hospitalization
Major Surgical Pack
Induce Anesthesia
Torbugesic
Fentanyl Patch
Diaphragmatic Hernia
Office Call
Standard O.R. Setup
ECG Monitoring
Complete Blood Count (CBC)
Biochemistry Profile
Radiograph—1st
Additional Radiograph
Isoflurane (First 20 min)
Isoflurane (Add'l 20 min)
IV Catheter & Insertion
Lactated Ringer's Solution
Administration Set
Hospitalization
Diaphragmatic Hernia Repair
Amoxicillin 400 mg. tabs
Amoxi—Inject
Prednisone Injection
Gavage (per liter)
Torbugesic
Major Surgical Pack
Assistant Technician (hourly)
Induce Anesthesia
Rimadyl
Disc—Minor
Office Call
Radiograph—1st
Additional Radiograph
IV Catheter & Insertion
Hospitalization
Prednisone 20 mg. tabs
Dexamethasone Sodium Phosphate
Isoflurane (First 20 min)
Preanesthetic Screen
Doxorubicin
Doxorubicin—10 mg.
IV Catheter & Insertion
Administration Set
Saline Solution (0.9% NaCl)
Ear Ablation—Bilateral
Office Call
Isoflurane (First 20 min)
Isoflurane (Add'l 20 min)
IV Catheter & Insertion
Lactated Ringer's Solution
Administration Set
Ear Ablation—Bilateral
Amoxicillin 400 mg. tabs
Amoxi—Inject
Prednisone 5 mg. tabs
Prednisone Injection

Oti-Clens
Gentocin Otic/DMSO
Bacterial Culture/Sensitivity
Flush and/or Curette Ears
ECG Monitoring
Standard O.R. Setup
Preanesthetic Screen
3M C/C Med Collar—Size 30
Major Surgical Pack
Induce Anesthesia
Torbugesic
Fentanyl Patch
Ear Ablation—Unilateral
Office Call
Isoflurane (First 20 min)
Isoflurane (Add'l 20 min)
IV Catheter & Insertion
Lactated Ringer's Solution
Administration Set
Ear Ablation—Unilateral
Amoxicillin 400 mg. tabs
Amoxi—Inject
Prednisone 5 mg. tabs
Prednisone Injection
Oti-Clens
Gentocin Otic/DMSO
Bacterial Culture/Sensitivity
Flush and/or Curette Ears
ECG Monitoring
Standard O.R. Setup
Preanesthetic Screen
3M C/C Med Collar—Size 30
Radiograph—1st
Additional Radiograph
Major Surgical Pack
Ear Swab Smear—Microscope Exam
Induce Anesthesia
Torbugesic
Fentanyl Patch
Ear Crop
ECG Monitoring
Isoflurane (First 20 min)
Ear Crop
Microchip Insertion
Preanesthetic Screen
Bandage—Small
Induce Anesthesia
Major Surgical Pack
Torbugesic
Fentanyl Patch
Emergency Protocol
(first night only)
Office Call
Emergency Call
IV Catheter & Insertion
Administration Set

Lactated Ringer's Mix
Oxygen Therapy
Dexamethasone SP
ECG—Routine
Complete Blood Count (CBC)
Biochemistry Profile
Radiograph—1st
Additional Radiograph
Cephalothin Sodium Inj.
Hospitalization
Torbugesic
Entropion—Bilateral
Office Call
Standard O.R. Setup
ECG Monitoring
Isoflurane (First 20 min)
Isoflurane (Add'l 20 min)
Hospitalization
Entropion—Bilateral
BNPH
3M C/C Med Collar—Size 30
Preanesthetic Screen
Major Surgical Pack
Induce Anesthesia
Torbugesic
Fentanyl Patch
Entropion—Unilateral
Office Call
Standard O.R. Setup
ECG Monitoring
Isoflurane (First 20 min)
Isoflurane (Add'l 20 min)
Hospitalization
Entropion Single
BNPH
3M C/C Med Collar—Size 30
Preanesthetic Screen
Major Surgical Pack
Induce Anesthesia
Torbugesic
Fentanyl Patch
Enucleation
Office Call
Standard O.R. Setup
ECG Monitoring
Isoflurane (First 20 min)
Isoflurane (Add'l 20 min)
IV Catheter & Insertion
Lactated Ringer's Solution
Administration Set
Enucleation
Amoxicillin 400 mg. tabs
Amoxi—Inject
Preanesthetic Screen
3M C/C Med Collar—Size 30
Hospitalization

Major Surgical Pack
Induce Anesthesia
Torbugesic
Fentanyl Patch
Ethylene Glycol Toxicity
Office Call
Administration Set
IV Catheter & Insertion
Lactated Ringer's Solution
Ethonal Administration
Hospitalization
Apomorphine Injection
Charcoal Administration
Complete Blood Count (CBC)
Biochemistry Profile
Urinalysis/Sediment Exam
Feline Urological Syndrome
Office Call
ECG Monitoring
Relieve Urinary Obstruction
Indwelling Urinary Catheter
Urinalysis/Sediment Exam
Complete Blood Count (CBC)
Biochemistry Profile
Feline Leukemia Test (Inhouse)
Radiograph—1st
Isoflurane (First 20 min)
Isoflurane (Add'l 20 min)
IV Catheter & Insertion
Saline Solution (0.9% NaCl)
Administration Set
Hospitalization
S/D FELINE 10#
Amoxi—Inject
Prednisone Injection
BUN
Creatinine
Amoxicillin 100 mg. tabs
Additional Radiograph
Feline Urological Syndrome—Minor
Office Call
Urinalysis/Sediment Exam
Amoxi—Inject
Prednisone Injection
Radiograph—1st
Medicate/Boarding (Cat)
S/D FELINE 10#
Amoxicillin 100 mg. tabs
Additional Radiograph
Biochemistry Profile
Complete Blood Count (CBC)
Feline Vax Bundle
Wellness Exam
FELV (Annual)
FVRCCP (Annual)
1 yr. Feline Rabies

Fecal Flotation

Femoral Head Removal—Canine
Office Call
Standard O.R. Setup
ECG Monitoring
Radiograph—1st
Additional Radiograph
Isoflurane (First 20 min)
Isoflurane (Add'l 20 min)
IV Catheter & Insertion
Lactated Ringer's Solution
Administration Set
Femoral Head & Neck Resect (K-9)
Preanesthetic Screen
Hospitalization
Major Surgical Pack
Induce Anesthesia
Torbugesic
Fentanyl Patch

Femoral Head Removal—Feline
Office Call
Standard O.R. Setup
ECG Monitoring
Isoflurane (First 20 min)
Isoflurane (Add'l 20 min)
IV Catheter & Insertion
Lactated Ringer's Solution
Administration Set
Femoral Head & Neck (Feline)
Preanesthetic Screen
Hospitalization
Major Surgical Pack
Amoxi—Inject
Torbugesic
Torb-VAL Suspension

Gastric Torsion
Office Call
Standard O.R. Setup
Emergency Call
Gastric Lavage
Complete Blood Count (CBC)
Biochemistry Profile
ECG Monitoring
Torbugesic
Isoflurane(First 20 min)
Isoflurane (Add'l 20 min)
IV Catheter & Insertion
Lactated Ringer's Mix
Administration Set
Hospitalization
Gastropexy
I/D CAN 1459/2918
I/D 20#
Banamine Injection
Dexemethasone Sodium Posphate
Betadine Saline 250 cc

Atropine Inj.
Cephalothin Sodium Inj.
Cephalexin 500 mg.
Fentanyl Patch

Gastrotomy
Office Call
Standard O.R. Setup
ECG Monitoring
Complete Blood Count (CBC)
Biochemistry Profile
Radiograph—1st
Additional Radiograph
Gastrointestinal X-ray Series
Barium Administration
Isoflurane (First 20 min)
Isoflurane (Add'l 20 min)
IV Catheter & Insertion
Lactated Ringer's Solution
Administration Set
Gastrotomy
I/D CAN 1459/2918
Amoxicillin 400 mg. tabs
Amoxi—Inject
Hospitalization
Induce Anesthesia
Major Surgical Pack
Torbugesic
Fentanyl Patch

Geriatric Physical—Large
Office Call
Complete Blood Count (CBC)
Biochemistry Profile
Urinalysis/Sediment Exam
Abdomen (2 views)
Thorax (2 views)
Fecal Flotation
ECG—Routine
Thyroxine—Free T4
SPECIAL DISCOUNT

Geriatric Physical—Small
Complete Blood Count (CBC)
Biochemistry Profile
Radiograph—first view
Additional Radiograph
Urinalysis/Sediment Exam
ECG—Routine
Office Call
Fecal Flotation
Thyroxine-Free T4
SPECIAL DISCOUNT

Hematoma—Major
Office Call
Standard O.R. Setup
ECG Monitoring
Flush and/or Curette Ears
Isoflurane (First 20 min)

Isoflurane (Add'l 20 min)
Hematoma Ear Surgery—Major
Amoxicillin 400 mg. tabs
Amoxi—Inject
Prednisone Injection
Otomax 15 ml
Bacterial Culture/Sensitivity
Preanesthetic Screen
Hospitalization
Ear Swab Smear—Microscope Exam
Major Surgical Pack
Pain Management

Hematoma—Tube
Office Call
Standard O.R. Setup
ECG Monitoring
Flush and/or Curette Ears
Isoflurane (First 20 min)
Isoflurane (Add'l 20 min)
Hematoma Ear Surgery—Tube
Amoxicillin 400 mg. tabs
Amoxi—Inject
Prednisone Injection
Otomax 15 ml
Bacterial Culture/Sensitivity
Preanesthetic Screen
Ear Swab Smear—Microscope Exam
Major Surgical Pack
Hospitalization
Pain Management

Insect Bite
Office Call
Amoxicillin 400 mg. tabs
Amoxi—Inject
Diphenhydramine 50 mg.
Diphenhydramine Injection
Prednisone Injection
Epinephrine

Intestinal Anastomosis
Office Call
Radiograph—1st
Additional Radiograph
Standard O.R. Setup
Hospitalization
Intestinal Anastomosis
I/D 20#
Cephalothin Sodium Inj.
Cephalexin 500 mg.
Isoflurane (First 20 min)
Isoflurane (Add'l 20 min)
ECG Monitoring
Preanesthetic Screen
IV Catheter & Insertion
Administration Set
Lactated Ringer's Mix
Gavage (per liter)

IV Pump Fee
Torbugesic
Induce Anesthesia
Major Surgical Pack
Pain Management

Isoflurane
Isoflurane (First 20 min)
Isoflurane (Add'l 20 min)
Preanesthetic Screen
ECG Monitoring
Induce Anesthesia

IV Fluids
IV Catheter & Insertion
Administration Set
Lactated Ringer's Solution
IV Pump Fee

Knee Surgery-MPL/LPL
Office Call
Standard O.R. Setup
ECG Monitoring
Robert Jones Bandage—Med.
Radiograph—1st
Additional Radiograph
Isoflurane (First 20 min)
Isoflurane (Add'l 20 min)
IV Catheter & Insertion
Lactated Ringer's Solution
Administration Set
Hospitalization
Repair Patellar Luxation
Amoxicillin 400 mg. tabs
Amoxi—Inject
Preanesthetic Screen
Major Surgical Pack
Induce Anesthesia
Pain Management

Mastectomy
Office Call
Complete Blood Count (CBC)
Biochemistry Profile
Radiograph—1st
Additional Radiograph
Urinalysis/Sediment Exam
ECG—Routine
ECG Monitoring
Isoflurane (First 20 min)
Isoflurane (Add'l 20 min)
IV Catheter & Insertion
Administration Set
Lactated Ringer's Mix
Cephalothin Sodium Inj.
Hospitalization
Cephalexin 500 mg.
Histopathology: 1–5 Specimens
Standard O.R. Setup
Mastectomy

Major Surgical Pack
Bandage—Small
Induce Anesthesia
Torbugesic
Fentanyl Patch
Ophthalmic Exam
Office Call
Stain Eye
Shirmer Tear Test
Pressure
Oronasal Fistula—K9—Bilateral
Office Call
Standard O.R. Setup
ECG Monitoring
Isoflurane (First 20 min)
Isoflurane (Add'l 20 min)
IV Catheter & Insertion
Lactated Ringer's Solution
Administration Set
Oronasal Fistula—Bilateral
Amoxicillin 400 mg. tabs
Amoxi—Inject
Preanesthetic Screen
Induce Anesthesia
Hospitalization
Fluoride Treatment
Major Surgical Pack
Pain Management
Oronasal Fistula—K9—Single
Office Call
Standard O.R. Setup
ECG Monitoring
Isoflurane (First 20 min)
Isoflurane (Add'l 20 min)
IV Catheter & Insertion
Lactated Ringer's Solution
Administration Set
Canine Scale & Polish—Average
Oronasal Fistula—Dbl flap
Amoxicillin 400 mg. tabs
Amoxi—Inject
Preanesthetic Screen
Fluoride Treatment
Hospitalization
Major Surgical Pack
Induce Anesthesia
Pain Management
Oronasal Fistula—Feline
Office Call
Standard O.R. Setup
ECG Monitoring
Isoflurane (First 20 min)
Isoflurane (Add'l 20 min)
IV Catheter & Insertion
Lactated Ringer's Solution
Administration Set

Feline Scale & Polish
Oronasal Fistula Minor
Amoxicillin 100 mg. tabs
Amoxi—Inject
Preanesthetic Screen
Hospitalization
Fluoride Treatment
Major Surgical Pack
Induce Anesthesia
Pain Management
Otitis
Office Call
ECG Monitoring
Flush &/or Curette Ears
Bacterial Culture/Sensitivity
Isoflurane (First 20 min)
Isoflurane (Add'l 20 min)
Amoxicillin 400 mg. tabs
Amoxi—Inject
Prednisone 20 mg. tabs
Prednisone Injection
Liquichlor ½ oz.
Oti-Clens
Preanesthetic Screen
Ear Swab Smear—Microscope Exam
Induce Anesthesia
Parvo—First Day
Office Call
Complete Blood Count—(CBC)
Parvo Virus Test
IV Catheter & Insertion
Lactated Ringer's Mix
Administration Set
Hospitalization
Cephalothin Sodium Inj.
Banamine Injection
Dexamethasone Sodium Phosphate
Endoserum (per cc)
Chlorpromazine Injection
Additional Injection
Hetastarch
Parvo—Add'l Days
Hospitalization
Lactated Ringer's Mix
Cephalothin Sodium Inj.
Chlorpromazine Injection
Additional Injection
Administration Set
Hetastarch
Perineal Hernia—Bilateral
Office Call
Complete Blood Count (CBC)
Biochemistry Profile
Radiograph—1st
Additional Radiograph
Isoflurane (First 20 min)

Isoflurane (Add'l 20 min)
IV Catheter & Insertion
Lactated Ringer's Solution
Administration Set
Hospitalization
ECG Monitoring
Standard O.R. Setup
Cephalothin Sodium Inj.
Cephalexin 500 mg.
Torbugesic
3M C/C Med Collar—Size 30
Major Surgical Pack
Induce Anesthesia
Rimadyl

Perineal Hernia—Single
Office Call
Complete Blood Count (CBC)
Biochemistry Profile
Radiograph—1st
Additional Radiograph
Isoflurane (First 20 min)
Isoflurane (Add'l 20 min)
IV Catheter & Insertion
Lactated Ringer's Solution
Administration Set
Hospitalization
Perineal Hernia—Single
ECG Monitoring
Standard O.R. Setup
Cephalothin Sodium Inj.
Cephalexin 500 mg.
Torbugesic
3M C/C Med Collar—Size 30
Major Surgical Pack
Induce Anesthesia
Rimadyl

Proptosed Eye
Office Call
Standard O.R. Setup
ECG Monitoring
Isoflurane (First 20 min)
Eye Surgery
Tarsorrophy & 3rd Eyelid Flap
Chloramphenicol 250 mg. tabs
Chloramphenicol Injection
Banamine Injection
Dexamethasone Sodium Phosphate
Preanesthetic Screen
Gentocin Ophthalmic Solution
Hospitalization
Induce Anesthesia
Minor Surgical Pack
IV Catheter & Insertion
Lactated Ringer's Solution
Torbugesic
Torb-VAL Suspension

Pyometra
Office Call
Standard O.R. Setup
ECG Monitoring
Complete Blood Count (CBC)
Biochemistry Profile
Radiograph—1st
Additional Radiograph
Isoflurane (First 20 min)
Isoflurane (Add'l 20 min)
IV Catheter & Insertion
Lactated Ringer's Solution
Administration Set
IV Pump Fee
Hospitalization
Pyometra
Amoxicillin 400 mg. tabs
Amoxi—Inject
Banamine Injection
Major Surgical Pack
Induce Anesthesia

Root Canal
Dental Radiographs—1 thru 5
Isoflurane (First 20 min)
Isoflurane (Add'l 20 min)
Root Canal—PM4
Amoxi—Inject
Amoxicillin 400 mg. tabs

Salivary Gland Removal
Office Call
Standard O.R. Setup
ECG Monitoring
Cytology—Lab
Isoflurane (First 20 min)
Isoflurane (Add'l 20 min)
IV Catheter & Insertion
Lactated Ringer's Solution
Administration Set
IV Pump Fee
Drain Tube(s)
Salivary Cyst
Amoxicillin 400 mg. tabs
Amoxi—Inject
Prednisone Injection
Panalog 15 ml
Preanesthetic Screen
Hospitalization
Major Surgical Pack
Induce Anesthesia
Pain Management

Seizures
Office Call
Urinalysis/Sediment Exam
Complete Blood Count (CBC)
Biochemistry Profile
ECG—Routine

Radiograph—1st
Additional Radiograph
Diazepam
IV Catheter & Insertion
Lactated Ringer's Solution
Administration Set
Phenobarbital 30 mg. tabs
Hospitalization
IV Pump Fee
Soft Palate
Office Call
Standard O.R. Setup
ECG Monitoring
Isoflurane (First 20 min)
Isoflurane (Add'l 20 min)
Oxygen Therapy
IV Catheter & Insertion
Lactated Ringer's Solution
Administration Set
Soft Palate Resection
Tonsillectomy
Stenotic Nares Repair
Amoxicillin 400 mg. tabs
Amoxi—Inject
Prednisone 20 mg. tabs
Prednisone Injection
Aminophylline Injection
Dopram-V Injection
Preanesthetic Screen
Hospitalization
Induce Anesthesia
Major Surgical Pack
Pain Management
Splenectomy
Office Call
Standard O.R. Setup
ECG Monitoring
Complete Blood Count (CBC)
Biochemistry Profile
Radiograph—1st
Additional Radiograph
Isoflurane (First 20 min)
Isoflurane (Add'l 20 min)
IV Catheter & Insertion
Lactated Ringer's Solution
Administration Set
IV Pump Fee
Hospitalization
Splenectomy
Amoxi—Inject
Banamine Injection
Histopathology: 1–5 Specimens
Packed Cell Volume (PCV)
Induce Anesthesia
Major Surgical Pack
Pain Management

Tail Amputation
Office Call
Standard O.R. Setup
ECG Monitoring
Isoflurane (first 20 min)
Isoflurane (Add'l 20 min)
Amputation—Tail
Amoxicillin 400 mg. tabs
Amoxi—Inject
Preanesthetic Screen
Bandage—Small
Induce Anesthesia
Major Surgical Pack
IV Catheter & Insertion
Lactated Ringer's Solution
Pain Management
Third Eyelid Flap
Office Call
Standard O.R. Setup
ECG Monitoring
Stain Eye
Isoflurane (First 20 min)
Third Eyelid Flap
Atropine Ophthalmic Drops
BNP
Preanesthetic Screen
3M C/C Med Collar—Size 30
Hospitalization
Induce Anesthesia
Minor Surgical Pack
Torn Nail
Office Call
Nail Trim
Bandage—Small
Isoflurane (First 20 min)
Clindamycin 150 mg.
Clindamycin Inj.
Prednisone Injection
ECG Monitoring
Preanesthetic Screen
Umbilical Hernia Repair
Office Call
Standard O.R. Setup
ECG Monitoring
Isoflurane (First 20 min)
Isoflurane (Add'l 20 min)
Umbilical Hernia Repair
Preanesthetic Screen
Hospitalization
Major Surgical Pack
Amoxi—Inject
Induce Anesthesia
IV Catheter & Insertion
Lactated Ringer's Solution

APPENDIX 3

More
Receptionist
Scripts

Telephone greeting:

Good Morning, ABC Animal Hospital, Mary speaking. How may I help you?

Client calls and asks to speak to doctor:

Mrs. Smith, can you please tell me the reason for your call? (Pet ill.) Can you describe what is going on with Baxter? That is a condition that Dr. Smith needs to see. Dr. Smith is in surgery now. I know you are concerned about Baxter. Dr. Smith can see Baxter this afternoon at 2, or will in the morning at 10 be a better time for you?

Recheck in two weeks:

After consultation the doctor notes on chart, Recheck in 2 weeks.

(At the time of billing client for services that day) Mrs. Smith, the doctor needs to recheck Fifi in two weeks. Is this day and time convenient for you?

(If client says she has to check her schedule at home.) "Mrs. Smith, when is the best time to call to set the appointment with you?" (At this time, enter a reminder to come up for the day you are to call Mrs. Smith.)

What to say when you get the answering machine:

Hello, this is Mary, calling from ABC Animal Hospital; Dr. Smith needs to see Baxter for a recheck on Friday. Please give me a call at _____ to schedule a time for you to bring in Baxter. Thank you.

Shopper calls for price on dentals:

Mrs. Wilson, when was Fluffy's last visit with us? Oh, so Fluffy has never been to ABC Animal Hospital. I can tell you are concerned about Fluffy's teeth, but we are not able to give you a price over the telephone. We can schedule a time for Fluffy's teeth and gums to be examined by our nurse/technician. He/she will do a dental healthcare plan for Fluffy that includes the price. Tell me if Tuesday at 4 is good, or would you prefer a morning appointment?

Shopper calls for price on vaccines:

Mr. Roberts, are you an established client with ABC Animal Hospital? As an established client, we can get you in for a nursing pet protection appointment very economically. If you have not seen the doctor in a while, or have questions you want to ask the doctor specifically, we need to schedule you for a full doctor's consultation instead of the short nursing appointment. Which do you prefer to schedule?

Price:

The doctor's consultation with those services takes about twice as long, so we charge about twice as much. Which do you prefer to schedule today?

If not an established or preferred client: You can become a preferred client and take advantage of more economical services after the Annual Life Cycle Consultation. Let's go ahead and set that appointment for you right now.

Shopper calls for price on spays/neuters:

We are proud of the level of healthcare we deliver at ABC Animal Hospital. Our doctor will examine your pet and then give you an estimate of the cost. There are too many variables to consider giving you a price over the telephone.

I understand you want to have this surgery done as soon as possible. I will give our earliest consultation appointment for your convenience. Is Wednesday at 3 okay with you?

Client calls with "an emergency":

Remember to stay calm. Make sure you have the correct client and pet names to get the record ready. Establish from client what is happening with pet. Ask how soon they can bring in the pet. Alert the healthcare team that an emergency is on its way into the facility. Know your hospital policy in regard to payment for emergency services and paperwork that needs to be completed.

Reminder calls that vaccines are past due:

Mr. Brenn, this is Mary from ABC Animal Hospital. We are concerned about Rhett because his vaccine protection has expired. Can we schedule an appointment for him?

Call for missed appointment:

Mrs. Whitt, this is Betty calling from ABC Animal Hospital. Dr. Smith and I are concerned. Is everything okay at home? We missed seeing you and Fluffy for your appointment. Can we reschedule that now?

Missed appointment:

Dr. Smith and I were concerned about Fluffy. She had an appointment for 10:00 a.m. today. Is every thing OK at home? Would you like to reschedule for 4:30 p.m. today or 10:00 a.m. tomorrow?

Follow-up on visit:

Hi, Mrs. Jones, this is Jenny from the Animal Hospital. Dr. Smith and I wanted to make sure that Fluffy is OK after her visit yesterday. Any questions or problems that we didn't address that I can answer for you today? Any questions or problems, please don't hesitate to give me a call.

Follow-up on surgery:

Hi, Mrs. Jones, this is Patty from the Animal Hospital. Dr. Smith and I wanted to make sure that Fluffy is OK after yesterday's surgery. Does she seem uncomfortable at all?

How is her appetite today? Are you having any difficulty giving her the medication we sent home? Are there any questions or problems that we can answer for you? Any questions or problems, please don't hesitate to give me a call.

Follow-up on bath:

Hi, Mrs. Jones, this is Lani, the bather at the Animal Hospital. I just wanted to make certain that you were pleased with the results of Fluffy's bath yesterday. Any questions or problems, please don't hesitate to give me a call.

Follow-up on lab test:

Hi, Mrs. Jones, this is Cathy from the Animal Hospital. I have good news for you. We didn't identify any parasites on Figi's stool sample and her heartworm test also indicated that she doesn't have evidence of heartworm disease.

Follow-up on leukemia test:

Hi, Mrs. Jones, this is Vanessa from the Animal Hospital. As you may remember, we checked Spike for Feline Leukemia virus yesterday. Congratulations, at this point in time, Spike is free of Leukemia.

Follow-up on boarding:

Hi, Mrs. Jones, this is Alicia from the Animal Hospital. I just wanted to make certain that Ralph was happy to be at home after his stay at the resort.

Letter or card to send after three attempts to contact:

Dear Mrs. Smith,

Hope everything is doing well in the Smith Household. Dr. Jones and I have been trying to reach you to find out how Riya is doing after the visit with us last week.

We want to make sure that all of Riya's needs were met and that you didn't have any unanswered questions.

APPENDIX 4

More
Resort Forms

WHITE BOARD FOR GROOMING

PET NAME	Pick up time by owner	Pick up time by limo	Delivery time by limo	Cleansing bath	Medicated bath	Mitaban dip	Clip	Dematt			Ready to Go

*See medical record

✓ Indicates to be done by resort staff

✗ Indicates completed by resort staff

O Indicates to be done by grooming staff

● Indicates completed by grooming staff

WHITE BOARD FOR FOOD AND MEDICATION

PET NAME	MEDICATIONS & SPECIAL DIETS

RESORT GUEST LOCATION

1		10	19		28
2		11	20		29
3		12	21		30
4		13	22		31
5		14	23		32
6		15	24		33
7		16	25		34
8		17	26		35
9		18	27		36

The Pet Peabody: Boarding Policy and Fees

WELCOME ...

Thank you for boarding your pet at the **Pet Peabody**. Our enthusiastic staff will make every effort to see that your pet's stay is a happy one. The **Pet Peabody** is a member of the American Boarding Kennel Association and conforms to its strict standards of professional animal care. Our boarding facility is located adjacent to the Hankins Small Animal Clinic, thus assuring your pet of skilled veterinary care if needed.

BOARDING FEES

Boarding services are charged by the nmber of days your pet stays with us. If your pet is picked up prior to 9:00 a.m., you will not be charged for that day. Any dog staying over two days will be given a complimentary bath—the only exception being dogs picked up prior to 9:00 a.m. Unfortunately, we are unable to have our "guests" bathed, dried, and ready to go home before that time.

PET PEABODY HOURS

Monday thru Friday	8:00 AM – 5:30 PM
Saturday	8:00 AM – 5:00 PM
Sunday (Pickups only)	5:30 PM

OUR GOAL

Our goal is to make your pet as comfortable here as it would be in your own home. We welcome any of your questions, suggestions, or comments. And thank you for choosing the **Pet Peabody**—we really do care!

RATES and FEES: Summer 1994

For your pet's protection, all vaccines must be current. Bordetella—a specific kennel cough vaccine—is highly recommended. Your pet must be free of internal and external parasites. If not, treatment will be done at your expense. The **Pet Peabody** is not responsible for any personal belongings left with your pet.

OUR DELUXE Pet Peabody ACCOMMODATIONS INCLUDE ....

- Lodging in our specially designed suites or condos
- Feeding with *Science Diets* (or owner-provided food if you prefer)
- Fresh water served at all times
- Cleaning and sanitizing of individual pet quarters at least twice daily (more often if needed)

Especially for our Canine Guests .....

- Daily exercise in our **Pet Peabody** outdoor courtyard
- Heartworm preventative and vitamins administered according to your instructions
- Complimentary bath prior to discharge (if your dog stays with us over two days)

Especially for our Feline Friends

- Entertainment by our **Pet Peabody** in-house troupe of tropical fish
- Vitamins administered on schedule and according to your instructions

SAMPLE BOARDING POLICY

CARSON VALLEY KENNELS

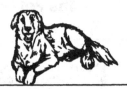

Thank you for choosing Carson Valley Kennels as your pet's "resort" destination. We can assure you that your pet will receive the best care from our professional staff. All climate-controlled runs are cleaned twice daily, our guests are let out individually once daily for 10 minutes to enjoy our exercise area, water bowls are sanitized and changed daily and our guests are fed Science Diet Maintenance. Our staff members have been trained to watch for any signs of discomfort while your pet vacations with us.

CHECK OUT TIME IS 10:00 AM

After 10:00 am you will be charged for that day's stay. Our charges begin on the first day your pet arrives, and for each day thereafter except the last day if you pick up before 10:00 am.

Our normal business hours are Monday through Sunday (7 days a week) 8 am to 5 pm. Special arrangements may be made for early or late arrivals or departures, please ask. Our holiday hours are 9 am to 10 am and 4 pm to 5 pm.

TOYS AND BONES

One toy will be accepted per pet. Please have your pets belongings permanently marked with your last name. We cannot be responsible for lost or chewed items.

TOWELS AND BEDDING

For sanitation all towels and bedding must be laundered daily. If you choose to leave bedding it will be laundered daily. Please have your bedding permanently marked with your last name.

We provide faux sheepskin "pup rugs" at no additional charge for your pets while they are with us. If it is more convenient for you to use our pup rug rather than your own, please be assured that it is laundered daily and your pet will be comfy. If your pet eats bedding or chews excessively please let us know. We cannot be responsible for chewed bedding or any medical problems caused to your pet from ingesting bedding when you have not asked that it be withheld.

FOOD

All our guests are fed twice daily unless otherwise specified by you. We feed Science Diet Maintenance. Please make us aware of any special feeding instructions.

If you prefer your pet be fed food which you bring, there is no additional charge. (It is actually more time consuming to feed individual special diets, but we will do it for you if it makes your pet more comfortable.)

To My Humans,

Best wishes from your grateful collie, Herman. When you decided to take me with you to Florida last week, I was thrilled. In my dreams I ran on white sunny beaches, sniffed sand crabs, plunged my paws deep in the warm surf.

Then you changed your mind. "He's a puppy; he might bark too much" you said.

I felt betrayed, abandoned, insulted …

But when you mentioned boarding me at the Pet Peabody, I perked up. "Neat name," I thought, "sounds sorta like 'doggie heaven.'" Little did I know!

As they escorted me to my Pet Peabody K-9 Kondo, I was immediately impressed with the musical barking of all the fine-looking dogs around me. Then the real fun began!!!

You see, this puppy has always dreamed of really letting go, of barking to my heart's content. Suddenly there it was – my dream come true! *Arf-arf! Arf-arf! AaaaWOOOOOO!* **BARK till you DROP!** It was **WONDERFUL!!!!**

Anyway, I'm a little hoarse from last night's Hallelujah Chorus but couldn't be happier. I'm well fed, well looked after – and well barked! **Please** stay in Florida as long as you like; life at the Pet Peabody is a blast!

Herman

The Pet Peabody
2604 West Jackson - Tupelo
The Vacation Destination for
   Your Favorite Pets

842-1119
(Adjacent to Hankins Small Animal Clinic)

TESTIMONIAL SAMPLE

Dear Pet Peabody:

That letter from Cinderella the Cat was a real tearjerker. Here's another one!

I'm a poodle. A **MALE** poodle. Until recently, my humans used to send me to a different groomer. I always returned from my grooming sessions so primped up and embarrassed that I would try to hide. Female dogs turned up their noses at me. Even the local kids would snicker.

When my humans started planning their latest trip, they decided to send me to the Pet Peabody. "Philippe, you'll love it," they told me. "The Pet Peabody is a very special place just for pets. Besides they have a **GREAT** groomer."

"Oh **NOOO!!!**," I thought, "She'll make me look like a doggie Dolly Parton!!!"

Imagine my surprise when I met Carla Hinds. She's the Pet Peabody groomer. Carla took one look at me and said, "Phillippe, from now on you're going to look like a dog, not a powder puff!"

"Cool!" I thought, wagging my tail, "I can **DEAL** with this lady!"

When Carla finished, I can modestly say I was a new animal. During that weekend, all the female dogs at the Pet Peabody started howling every time I walked by. Back in my neighborhood I'm treated with real respect. And guess what: I've even got a girlfriend. Several, in fact …

Thanks Pet Peabody; this is one pleased Poodle puppy!

Phillippe

ᴙᴙᴙ

Superb Pet Grooming
   By Carla Hinds
*2406 West Jackson Street

THE PET PEABODY
Call 842-1118 for Reservations
and Overnight Accommodations

*(Adjacent to Hankins Small Animal Clinic)

Dear Pet Peabody,

So why print all these doggie letters? I mean dogs are nice and everything, but all they basically do is wag their tails and say "Woof, Woof!" We cats are much more subtle—**AND** hard to please!

When my humans told me I was going to spend the weekend at the Pet Peabody, I said "Gimme a break!" I've been pampered all my life, and the thought of spending several days with a bunch of cats I don't even know nearly drove me crazy. What about my gourmet chow, my extra treats, my amusements? … **AND WHAT ABOUT MY TV SHOWS???** A cat of my quality simply can't be treated like the common herd.

I should have worried!

When they escorted me to my weekend Kat Kondo at the Pet Peabody, I was overwhelmed. ("Mmmmm…nice colors…this place is really cool," I thought.) The other cats around me appeared reassuringly distinguished. Then came the great chow, the personal attention, my special treats…**BUT WHAT ABOUT MY TV SHOWS???**

Suddenly I saw something in the center of the room. **FISH!!! … IN AN AQUARIUM!!** Wow, this is **BETTER** than TV!!!!!! All weekend I couldn't take my eyes off those gorgeous fish. Talk about kitty paradise!

On Sunday my humans came for me. Now we're back to (yawn) Monday night sports. I want my fish!!!

Thanks Pet Peabody!   **Matt the Cat**

The Pet Peabody
2604 West Jackson—Tupelo
Weekend Getaways for your
  Favorite Cats & Dogs

842-1119
(Adjacent to Hankins Small Animal Clinic)

Dear Humans,

     Greetings from Pierre, your peppy little party poodle. NEVER did I imagine that life at the Pet Peabody would be so much fun! Like any well-run resort, we have a regular schedule of tasty banquets, personalized groomings, community barkings, and pleasant strolls. I couldn't be happier. Now for the downside ....

     Remember the birthday party for your grandson? The one you gave just before leaving for LA? Remember how you laughed at my little pink poodle tongue lapping up leftover ice cream in the kitchen? Remember how I begged for birthday cake—and you gave it to me? And remember how "funny" you said I looked just before checking me into the Pet Peabody?

     You human talk about being "sick as a dog," but wait until YOU'RE the dog in question. Wait till you're miserable, friendless, and stuck in a strange place with the floor heaving and the walls spinning. Mother of All Poodles—was I a sick puppy!!!!!!

     Not to worry.

     The staff at the Pet Peabody was really cool. Within minutes I had not ONE but TWO veterinarians attending my every need. I'll SPARE you the gory details, but just be grateful you put me in a kennel next to the Hankins Small Animal Clinic. ALL of modern medicine was at my command!

     By surprise I would actually enjoy the resort atmosphere of the Pet Peabody once more. Thanks for sending me to such a great place—and one that's always prepared for the unexpected!

Pierre

Superb Pet Accommodations	**The Pet Peabody**
Weekends/Vacations	2604 W. Jackson
842-1119	Tupelo
Adjacent to Hankins Small Animal Clinic	

MEDICATIONS AND VETERINARY SERVICES

All medication is administered by our staff, according to your instructions. There is no additional charge for oral or topical medications. Injections are given by our medical staff at Carson Valley Veterinary Hospital for an additional $5.00 per day. Please be sure all medication is labeled correctly and the directions are clearly marked. Also, please include the phone number of your veterinarian in case of any health complications while you are away. If you would prefer we contact your veterinarian rather than Carson Valley Veterinary Hospital for emergencies, we will attempt to do so. Please make prior arrangements with them so they are aware of the circumstances.

The veterinarians at Carson Valley Veterinary Hospital are available 7 days a week to give vaccinations, exams, spays/neuters, dental care, or any special care your pet may need while staying with us. The client information card you signed gave permission for us to seek emergency care from these veterinarians. All payments for services must be made to Carson Valley Veterinary Hospital when picking up your pet.

GROOMING

We recommend baths for all dogs staying with us 3 days or longer. Although we completely clean the runs twice daily, spot clean periodically during the day, and launder bedding daily some guests are tidier than others. We like to send your pets home clean and smelling good. The Grooming Shop next door offers baths and special "hairdos." Please check with them for an appointment and their rates. If your pet is groomed, there will be no boarding charge for that pet the day of grooming. We offer baths only for short hair dogs. Our prices are $10 for dogs under 25#, $15 for 26–50#, and $20 for over 50#. If our staff does not feel your dog is a candidate for a bath only but needs attention from the groomer, we will let you know.

PLAYTIME AND PAMPERED PETS

All dogs are let out individually once daily into the exercise area and all cats are let out individually once daily into the cat play room for at least 10 minutes.
*For extra special pampering, we offer playtime, where your pet is taken out to play with a caring staff member so he/she can chase a ball, play with toys, or just get lots of praise and petting. This specialized pampering is in addition to the 10-minute exercise time all pets receive. Playtime lasts 15 minutes and costs an additional $3.00 per day.

Fifteen-minute walks on a leash in the field can be arranged. If you would like your pet to go on a walk with a staff member there will be an additional $3.00 charge per day per dog. We also require a signed release for this service.

BEDTIME

All dogs are given a "cookie" before bedtime. If your pet is on a special diet and cannot receive a treat, please let us know.

If you have any special requests please let us know; we will see what we can do. Please discuss any questions or concerns with Ann or Dianne. We appreciate your business and will do our best to provide your pet with a pleasurable stay.

SAMPLE CAGE CARD / REPORT CARD

FOLIO

CARSON VALLEY KENNEL

Towel	Diet	Med.	Exer.	Groom	Nails	Mdse.	PkUp	Delvy.	Train.	Vet.

REPORT CARD / RECORD

Begin: _____

EXERCISE

Name: _____ Rm: _____

Describe Pet:
_____

Describe Pet No. 2 _____

Special Instructions:
_____
_____
_____
_____
_____

1. _____   _____   _____
2. _____   _____   _____
3. _____   _____   _____
4. _____   _____   _____
5. _____   _____   _____
6. _____   _____   _____
7. _____   _____   _____
8. _____   _____   _____
9. _____   _____   _____
10. _____   _____   _____
11. _____   _____   _____
12. _____   _____   _____
13. _____   _____   _____
14. _____   _____   _____
15. _____   _____   _____
16. _____   _____   _____
17. _____   _____   _____
18. _____   _____   _____
19. _____   _____   _____
20. _____   _____   _____
21. _____   _____   _____
22. _____   _____   _____
23. _____   _____   _____
24. _____   _____   _____
25. _____   _____   _____
26. _____   _____   _____
27. _____   _____   _____
28. _____   _____   _____
29. _____   _____   _____
30. _____   _____   _____
31. _____   _____   _____

REPORT CARD / RECORD

Carson Valley Kennels   **Begin**_____

DIET RECORD

Name: _____   Rm: _____

Describe Pet: _____

Diet Food: _____

Food Location: _____

Feeding Times: 1st_____   2nd _____   3rd _____

Special Instructions _____

1. _____   _____   _____
2. _____   _____   _____
3. _____   _____   _____
4. _____   _____   _____
5. _____   _____   _____
6. _____   _____   _____
7. _____   _____   _____
8. _____   _____   _____
9. _____   _____   _____
10. _____   _____   _____
11. _____   _____   _____
12. _____   _____   _____
13. _____   _____   _____
14. _____   _____   _____
15. _____   _____   _____
16. _____   _____   _____
17. _____   _____   _____
18. _____   _____   _____
19. _____   _____   _____
20. _____   _____   _____
21. _____   _____   _____
22. _____   _____   _____
23. _____   _____   _____
24. _____   _____   _____
25. _____   _____   _____
26. _____   _____   _____
27. _____   _____   _____
28. _____   _____   _____
29. _____   _____   _____
30. _____   _____   _____
31. _____   _____   _____